Telemedicine Revolution
How to Take Control of Your Health Anytime. Anywhere

ife Success

Stories of Remote Doctor Visits

Erkan YILDIRIM

Table Of Contents

Chapter 1: Introduction to Telemedicine Revolution

What is Telemedicine?

Telemedicine is a revolutionary concept that is changing the way healthcare is delivered to patients all around the world. But what exactly is telemedicine? In simple terms, telemedicine refers to the use of technology, such as video calls or messaging, to provide remote healthcare services to patients. This means that you can consult with a doctor or healthcare provider from the comfort of your own home, office, or wherever you may be, without the need to physically visit a medical facility.

For busy professionals, telemedicine offers a flexible solution to their healthcare needs. Instead of taking time off work to visit a doctor's office, they can schedule a virtual consultation at a time that suits their busy schedule. This convenience allows them to prioritize their health without sacrificing valuable time at work. Similarly, tech-savvy individuals will appreciate the ease and convenience of telemedicine, as they are already comfortable using technology in their daily lives.

Individuals living in remote areas with limited access to healthcare facilities can greatly benefit from telemedicine consultations. Instead of traveling long distances to see a specialist, they can simply connect with a healthcare provider through a video call. This not only saves time and money on travel expenses but also ensures that they receive timely medical advice and treatment. Additionally, cost-conscious individuals may find telemedicine to be a more affordable option compared to traditional in-person visits, as it eliminates the need for transportation and other associated costs.

For parents of young children, telemedicine can be a convenient option for consultations regarding minor illnesses or routine checkups. Instead of dragging a sick child to a crowded waiting room, parents can seek medical advice from the comfort of their own home. Similarly, individuals with chronic conditions can benefit from regular telemedicine follow-up appointments with specialists, helping them manage their health more effectively. And for the elderly, telemedicine offers easier access to healthcare, allowing them to receive medical advice and treatment without the hassle of traveling to appointments. Overall, telemedicine is a game-changer in the healthcare industry, providing a convenient and cost-effective solution for individuals of all ages and backgrounds.

Benefits of Telemedicine

Telemedicine is revolutionizing the way people access healthcare, offering numerous benefits for a variety of individuals. For busy professionals, telemedicine provides a flexible solution to scheduling doctor appointments around their demanding work schedules. With remote consultations, they can easily fit in a quick check-up or discuss health concerns without having to take time off work or commute to a doctor's office. This convenience can save valuable time and reduce stress for those juggling multiple responsibilities. Tech-savvy individuals will appreciate the ease and convenience of telemedicine, as consultations can be conducted through video calls or messaging apps on their smartphones or computers. This modern approach to healthcare aligns with their comfort level with technology and allows them to take control of their health anytime, anywhere. By eliminating the need for in-person visits, telemedicine streamlines the healthcare process and makes it more accessible for those who prefer digital solutions.

For individuals living in remote areas with limited access to healthcare facilities, telemedicine offers a lifeline to medical consultations. By connecting with healthcare providers online, they can receive expert advice and treatment without the need to travel long distances. This can be especially beneficial for those in rural communities or areas lacking specialist care, ensuring they have access to the medical expertise they need to manage their health effectively. Cost-conscious individuals may find telemedicine to be a more affordable option compared to traditional in-person visits. With lower consultation fees and reduced travel expenses, telemedicine can help individuals save money on healthcare costs. By choosing telemedicine, they can receive quality medical care without breaking the bank, making it a practical choice for those looking to manage their health while staying within a budget.

Overall, telemedicine offers a range of benefits for various audiences, including parents of young children, individuals with chronic conditions, and the elderly. By embracing this innovative approach to healthcare, individuals can take charge of their health from anywhere, whether they are seeking minor illness consultations, regular follow up appointments, or easier access to healthcare services. With telemedicine, taking control of your health has never been more convenient or accessible.

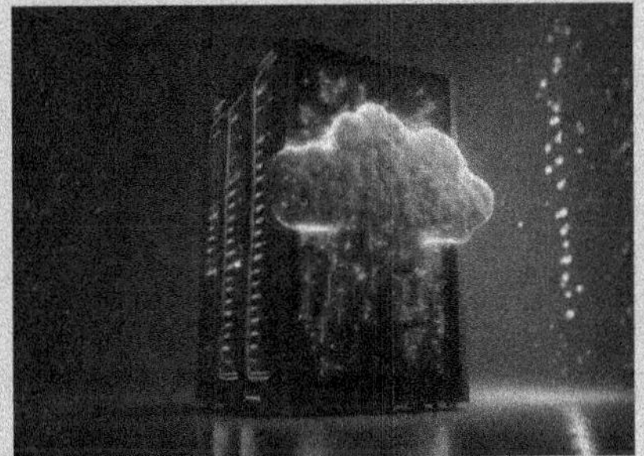

Evolution of Telemedicine

The evolution of telemedicine has been a game changer in the healthcare industry especially for busy professionals who struggle to find the time for traditional doctor appointments. With telemedicine, individuals can easily schedule consultations with healthcare providers from the comfort of their own home or office, eliminating the need to take time off work or deal with long wait times in a crowded waiting room. This flexibility allows busy professionals to prioritize their health without sacrificing their work commitments.

For tech savvy individuals, telemedicine offers a convenient and user friendly way to access healthcare services. With just a few clicks on a smartphone or computer, patients can connect with healthcare providers for virtual consultations, prescriptions, and follow up appointments. This seamless integration of technology into healthcare services makes it easier than ever for individuals to take control of their health anytime, anywhere.

Telemedicine also benefits those who are locationally challenged, such as individuals living in remote areas with limited access to healthcare facilities. With telemedicine, patients in rural or underserved areas can connect with healthcare providers without the need to travel long distances for in-person appointments. This increased access to healthcare services can greatly improve health outcomes for individuals who may otherwise struggle to receive timely medical care.

In addition to convenience and accessibility, telemedicine can also lead to cost savings for cost-conscious individuals. Virtual consultations often come at a lower price point compared to traditional in-person visits, making healthcare more affordable and accessible for individuals who are mindful of their healthcare expenses. By utilizing telemedicine services, individuals can receive quality healthcare without breaking the bank. Overall, the evolution of telemedicine has revolutionized the way individuals access healthcare services, offering a flexible, convenient, and cost-effective solution for busy professionals, tech-savvy individuals, those living in remote areas, and individuals who are mindful of their healthcare expenses. With the rise of telemedicine, individuals can take control of their health anytime, anywhere, without the constraints of traditional healthcare settings.

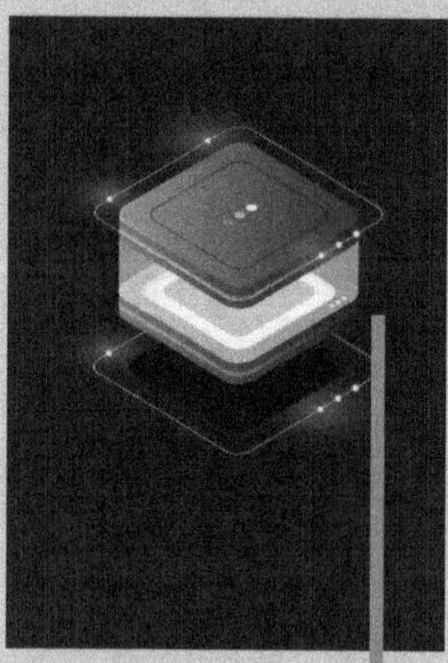

Understanding Telehealth vs Telemedicine

In today's fast-paced world, it can be challenging to find the time to prioritize our health. This is where telehealth and telemedicine come in as convenient solutions for busy professionals, tech-savvy individuals, and those living in remote areas with limited access to healthcare facilities. But what exactly is the difference between telehealth and telemedicine?

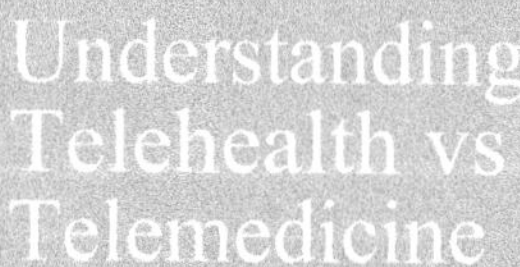

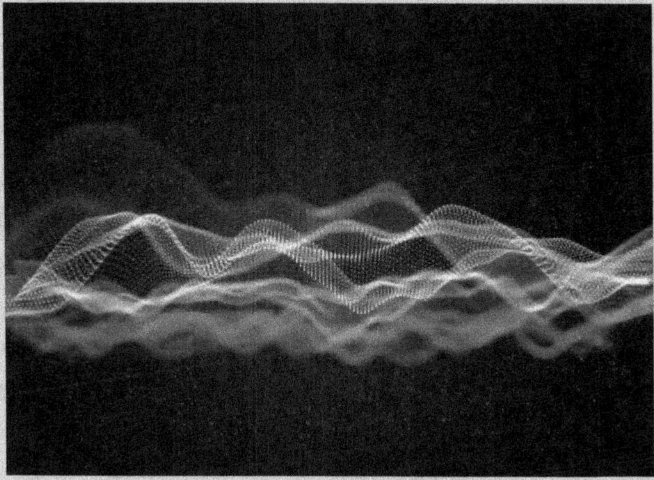

Telehealth is a broad term that encompasses a wide range of healthcare services delivered remotely through technology. This can include video consultations, remote monitoring of vital signs, and even virtual support groups. On the other hand, telemedicine specifically refers to the use of telecommunication technology to provide clinical healthcare services from a distance. This distinction is important to understand as it can help individuals navigate the various options available to them for remote healthcare.

For busy professionals who struggle to find time for in-person doctor appointments, telemedicine offers a flexible solution. By scheduling virtual consultations, individuals can receive the care they need without disrupting their work schedule. Similarly, tech-savvy individuals who are comfortable using technology will appreciate the ease and convenience of remote doctor visits. With just a few clicks, they can connect with a healthcare provider and get the guidance they need.

Individuals living in remote areas with limited access to healthcare facilities can also benefit from telemedicine consultations. By eliminating the need to travel long distances for appointments, telemedicine can help bridge the gap in healthcare disparities. Additionally, for cost-conscious individuals, telemedicine can potentially lead to lower healthcare costs compared to traditional in-person visits. This can be especially beneficial for those with chronic conditions who require regular follow-up appointments with specialists.

For parents of young children, telemedicine can be a convenient option for consultations regarding minor illnesses or checkups. Instead of rushing to the doctor's office with a sick child, parents can simply schedule a virtual visit from the comfort of their own home. Similarly, the elderly can also benefit from easier access to healthcare through telemedicine. For older adults who may have difficulty traveling for appointments, telemedicine offers a convenient alternative for receiving the care they need.

In conclusion, understanding the differences between telehealth and telemedicine is essential for individuals looking to take control of their health anytime, anywhere. Whether you are a busy professional, tech-savvy individual, or someone living in a remote area, telemedicine can offer a flexible and convenient solution for accessing healthcare services. By taking advantage of telemedicine, individuals can prioritize their health without sacrificing their busy schedules or breaking the bank.

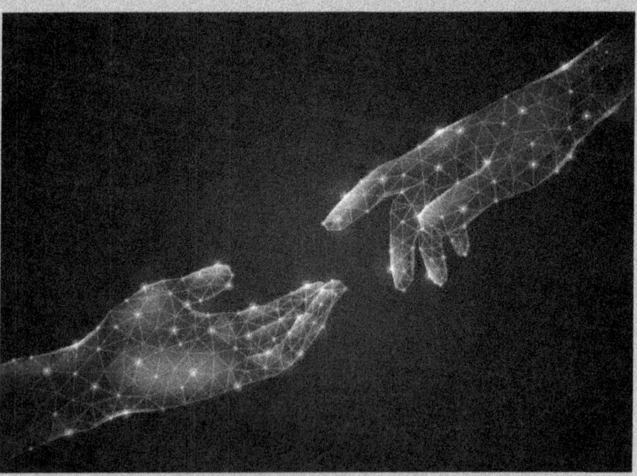

Telemedicine Revolution: How to Take Control of Your Health Anytime, Anywhere

Chapter 2: The Rise of Telemedicine

Growth of Telemedicine Industry

The growth of the telemedicine industry has been nothing short of remarkable in recent years. With advancements in technology and the increasing demand for convenient healthcare options, telemedicine has quickly become a popular choice for individuals looking to take control of their health anytime, anywhere. This subchapter will explore the various reasons why telemedicine has become a preferred option for busy professionals, tech-savvy individuals, those living in remote areas, and cost-conscious people.

Busy professionals, who often struggle to find time for doctor appointments due to their demanding schedules, can benefit greatly from telemedicine. With the ability to schedule remote consultations at their convenience, busy professionals can receive the medical care they need without having to take time off work. This flexibility is a game changer for individuals who are constantly on the go and need a more efficient way to manage their health.

Tech savvy individuals who are comfortable using technology in their daily lives will appreciate the ease and convenience of telemedicine. With just a few clicks on their smartphones or computers, they can connect with healthcare providers and receive expert medical advice without leaving their homes. This convenience is especially valuable for those who prefer digital solutions for various aspects of their lives, including healthcare.

For those living in remote areas with limited access to healthcare facilities, telemedicine consultations can be a lifesaver. Instead of traveling long distances to see a doctor, individuals in remote locations can simply log on to a telemedicine platform and receive the care they need from the comfort of their own homes. This increased access to healthcare can make a significant difference in the wellbeing of individuals who would otherwise struggle to receive timely medical attention.

Cost conscious people will also find telemedicine to be a cost effective alternative to traditional in person doctor visits. With lower consultation fees and reduced travel expenses, telemedicine can potentially lead to significant savings for individuals who are mindful of their healthcare spending. This financial benefit, combined with the convenience and accessibility of telemedicine, makes it an attractive option for those looking to take charge of their health without breaking the bank.

In conclusion, the growth of the telemedicine industry has opened up a world of possibilities for individuals seeking convenient, affordable, and accessible healthcare solutions. Whether you are a busy professional, a tech savvy individual, someone living in a remote area, or a cost conscious person, telemedicine offers a flexible and efficient way to take control of your health anytime, anywhere. By embracing the benefits of telemedicine, you can ditch the waiting room and empower yourself to prioritize your health in a way that fits seamlessly into your busy lifestyle.

Telemedicine Technologies

Telemedicine has revolutionized the way healthcare is delivered, offering a convenient and efficient solution for individuals with busy schedules. With telemedicine technologies, busy professionals can now easily schedule virtual consultations with their healthcare providers without having to take time off work for in person appointments. This flexibility allows individuals to take control of their health anytime, anywhere, making it easier to prioritize their well being even amidst hectic schedules.

For tech savvy individuals, telemedicine technologies offer a seamless and user friendly experience for remote doctor visits. From video consultations to secure messaging platforms, telemedicine platforms are designed to cater to individuals comfortable using technology. This ease and convenience of accessing healthcare services remotely can empower tech savvy individuals to stay proactive about their health and seek medical advice whenever needed.

Individuals living in remote areas with limited access to healthcare facilities can greatly benefit from telemedicine consultations. By leveraging telemedicine technologies, locationally challenged individuals can connect with healthcare providers virtually, eliminating the need for long travel distances to see a doctor. This accessibility to healthcare services can help bridge the gap in healthcare disparities, ensuring that everyone has equal opportunities to receive quality medical care regardless of their geographical location.

Cost conscious individuals can also appreciate the potential cost savings associated with telemedicine compared to traditional in person visits. With telemedicine technologies, individuals can avoid unnecessary expenses such as transportation costs and missed work hours. This cost effective solution allows individuals to seek medical advice and treatment without breaking the bank, making healthcare more affordable and accessible for those looking to manage their expenses efficiently.

In conclusion, telemedicine technologies are a game-changer for various demographics, including parents of young children, individuals with chronic conditions, and the elderly. By embracing telemedicine, individuals can take charge of their health from anywhere, benefiting from the convenience, accessibility, and cost savings offered by remote healthcare consultations. Whether you're a busy professional, a tech-savvy individual, or someone living in a remote location, telemedicine technologies empower you to prioritize your health and well-being without compromising on your daily commitments.

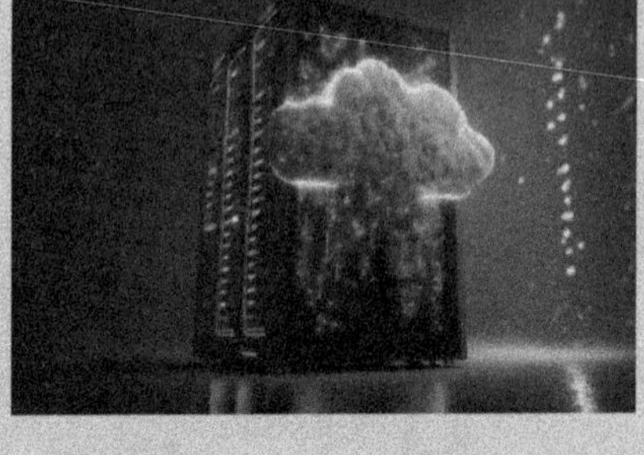

Telemedicine Regulations and Policies

In recent years, telemedicine has emerged as a convenient and efficient way for individuals to access healthcare services from the comfort of their own homes. However, with this new technology comes a need for regulations and policies to ensure that patients are receiving high-quality care and that healthcare providers are practicing ethically and responsibly.

One of the key regulations governing telemedicine is the Health Insurance Portability and Accountability Act (HIPAA), which protects the privacy and security of patients' medical information. Telemedicine providers must comply with HIPAA regulations to ensure that patients' sensitive health data is kept confidential and secure. Additionally, many states have their own regulations regarding telemedicine, including requirements for licensure, informed consent, and reimbursement policies.

When it comes to reimbursement for telemedicine services, policies vary depending on the state and insurance provider. Some states have parity laws that require insurance companies to cover telemedicine services at the same rate as in-person visits while others may have restrictions or limitations on reimbursement for virtual consultations. It is important for patients to understand their insurance coverage and the policies of their healthcare providers when considering telemedicine as an option for medical care.

For healthcare providers, there are also regulations and policies in place to ensure that they are practicing telemedicine ethically and responsibly. This includes guidelines for prescribing medications, conducting virtual examinations, and maintaining accurate medical records. Providers must also be licensed in the state where the patient is located in order to deliver telemedicine services legally.

Overall, telemedicine regulations and policies are constantly evolving as technology advances and more individuals turn to virtual healthcare options. It is important for both patients and healthcare providers to stay informed about the latest regulations and policies governing telemedicine to ensure that they are receiving and delivering high quality care in a safe and secure manner. As telemedicine continues to revolutionize the healthcare industry, adhering to these regulations and policies will be crucial in ensuring the success and sustainability of remote healthcare services for individuals across all demographics.

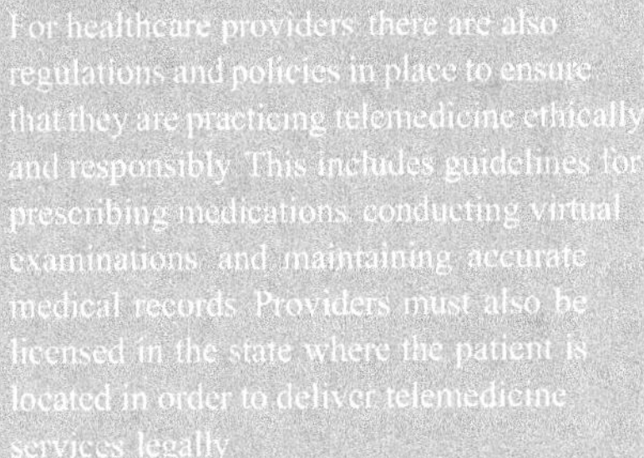

Telemedicine Adoption Rates

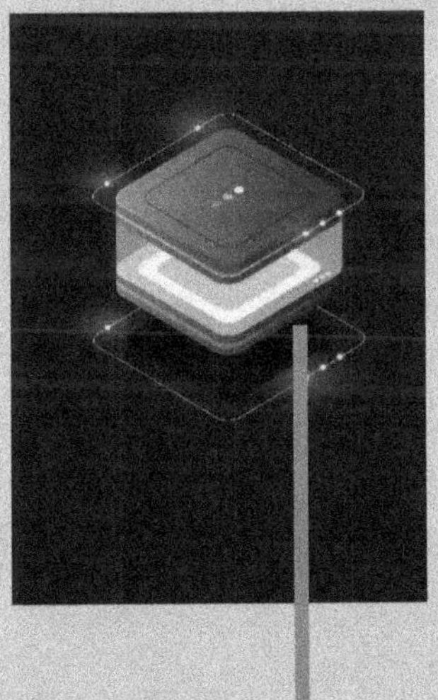

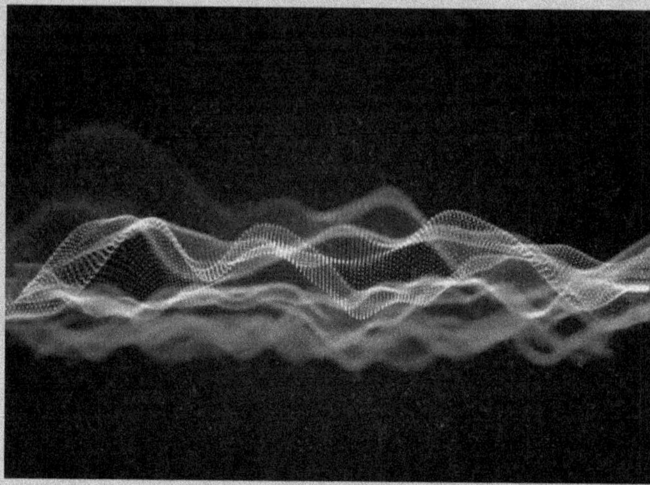

Telemedicine adoption rates have been steadily increasing in recent years, and for good reason. This innovative approach to healthcare offers a flexible and convenient solution for individuals with demanding schedules, such as busy professionals. These individuals often struggle to find the time to take off work for traditional in-person doctor appointments. With telemedicine, consultations can be easily conducted remotely, saving time and reducing the need for travel.

Tech-savvy individuals are also embracing telemedicine as a convenient way to access healthcare services. Those comfortable using technology will appreciate the ease of scheduling remote doctor visits and the convenience of consulting with healthcare professionals from the comfort of their own homes. Telemedicine allows for quick and efficient communication between patients and providers, making it a popular choice for those who value convenience and efficiency.

For those living in remote areas with limited access to healthcare facilities, telemedicine can be a lifesaver. These locationally challenged individuals may have difficulty accessing traditional in-person care, making telemedicine consultations a valuable alternative. By utilizing telemedicine services, individuals in remote areas can receive the healthcare they need without the added stress of traveling long distances to see a doctor.

Telemedicine Revolution: How to Take Control of Your Health Anytime, Anywhere

Cost conscious individuals are also turning to telemedicine as a way to potentially lower their healthcare costs Telemedicine consultations are often more affordable than traditional in person visits making them an attractive option for those looking to save money on healthcare expenses By choosing telemedicine individuals can receive quality healthcare services without breaking the bank

In conclusion telemedicine adoption rates are on the rise and for good reason This innovative approach to healthcare offers a flexible and convenient solution for a wide range of individuals including busy professionals tech savvy individuals those living in remote areas and cost conscious individuals By embracing telemedicine individuals can take control of their health anytime anywhere and enjoy the benefits of quick and efficient remote consultations with healthcare professionals

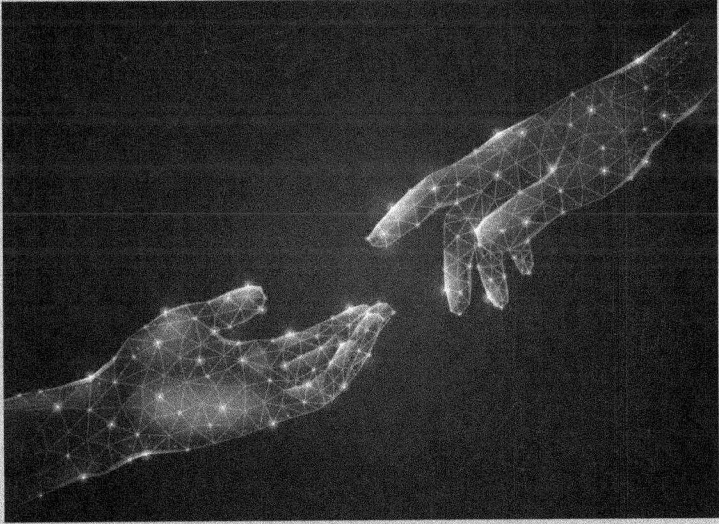

Telemedicine Revolution: How to Take Control of Your Health Anytime, Anywhere

Chapter 3: Telemedicine Tools and Resources

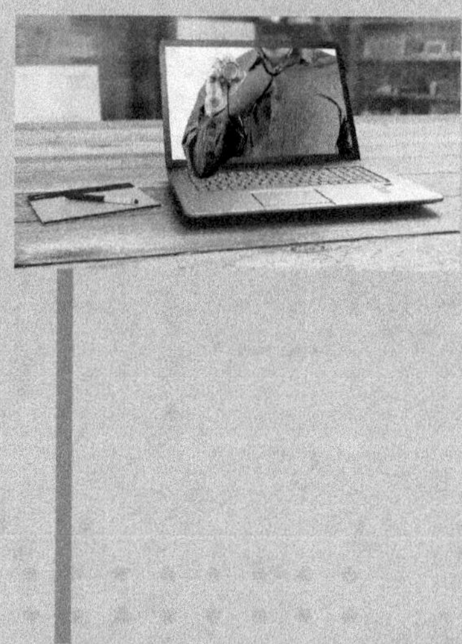

Telemedicine Platforms and Apps

Telemedicine platforms and apps are revolutionizing the way individuals receive healthcare services. For busy professionals who struggle to find time for doctor appointments due to demanding schedules, telemedicine offers a flexible solution. With the ability to consult with healthcare providers remotely, busy professionals can save time and receive the care they need without disrupting their work commitments. Tech savvy individuals will appreciate the ease and convenience of telemedicine platforms and apps. These individuals are comfortable using technology and will find it convenient to schedule and attend remote doctor visits. With just a few clicks on their smartphones or computers, they can connect with healthcare providers and receive medical advice or prescriptions from the comfort of their own homes.

For those living in remote areas with limited access to healthcare facilities, telemedicine consultations can be a lifesaver. Telemedicine bridges the gap between patients and healthcare providers, allowing individuals in remote locations to receive medical advice and treatment without the need to travel long distances. This is especially beneficial for individuals in rural areas who may struggle to access quality healthcare services. Cost-conscious people will appreciate the potential savings that telemedicine can offer compared to traditional in-person visits. With telemedicine, individuals can avoid costly hospital or clinic visits for minor illnesses or routine checkups. This can lead to lower healthcare costs overall, making it a more affordable option for those looking to manage their health without breaking the bank.

In conclusion, telemedicine platforms and apps are a game-changer for individuals in various situations, including busy professionals, tech-savvy individuals, those living in remote areas, and cost-conscious individuals. Additionally, telemedicine can also benefit parents of young children, individuals with chronic conditions, and the elderly by offering convenient access to healthcare services. With the convenience and flexibility that telemedicine provides, individuals can take control of their health anytime, anywhere.

Connecting with Healthcare Providers Online

In today's fast-paced world, finding the time to visit a healthcare provider can be a challenge for many individuals. Whether you're a busy professional with a demanding schedule, a tech-savvy individual who values convenience, or someone living in a remote area with limited access to healthcare facilities, telemedicine offers a flexible solution for connecting with healthcare providers online. By taking advantage of telemedicine, you can take control of your health anytime, anywhere.

For busy professionals, telemedicine provides a convenient alternative to traditional in-person doctor appointments. Instead of taking time off work to visit a healthcare provider, you can schedule a remote consultation at a time that works for you. This flexibility allows you to prioritize your health without disrupting your busy schedule. With telemedicine, you can easily connect with healthcare providers online, saving time and reducing the stress of fitting appointments into your already packed calendar.

Tech-savvy individuals will appreciate the ease and convenience of telemedicine consultations. By using technology to connect with healthcare providers online, you can access quality care without the hassle of scheduling and traveling to in-person appointments. Whether you prefer video calls, phone consultations, or secure messaging, telemedicine offers a variety of communication options to suit your preferences. With just a few clicks, you can connect with a healthcare provider and receive the care you need from the comfort of your own home.

For those living in remote areas with limited access to healthcare facilities, telemedicine can be a lifesaver. By connecting with healthcare providers online, you can access quality care without the need to travel long distances for in-person appointments. This can be especially beneficial for individuals with chronic conditions who require regular follow-up appointments with specialists. With telemedicine, you can receive the care you need without the added stress and expense of traveling to a healthcare facility.

In addition to convenience and accessibility, telemedicine can also help you save money on healthcare costs. By opting for remote consultations instead of traditional in-person visits, you can potentially lower your healthcare expenses. This cost-saving benefit makes telemedicine an attractive option for individuals who are looking to take control of their health without breaking the bank. Whether you're a cost-conscious individual or simply looking for a more affordable healthcare option, telemedicine can help you manage your health without sacrificing quality care.

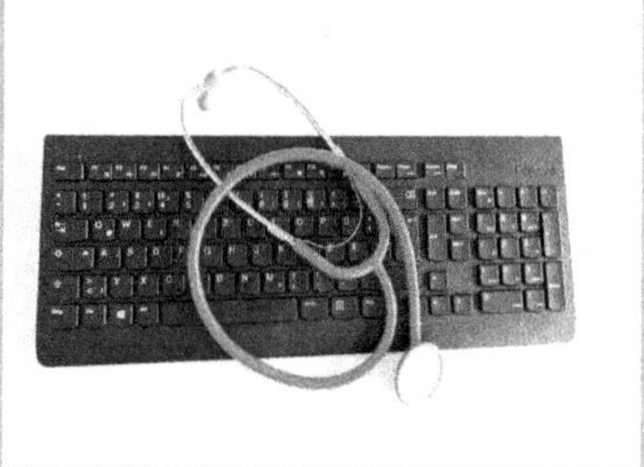

Virtual Consultations and Remote Monitoring

Virtual consultations and remote monitoring are revolutionizing the way we access healthcare, providing a convenient and efficient solution for busy professionals who struggle to find time for in-person doctor appointments. With telemedicine, individuals can schedule consultations at their convenience, eliminating the need to take time off work or travel to a medical facility. This flexibility allows for seamless integration of healthcare into even the busiest of schedules, ensuring that no one has to compromise their health due to time constraints.

For tech-savvy individuals who are comfortable using technology, telemedicine offers a user-friendly and convenient way to connect with healthcare providers. Through virtual consultations, patients can discuss their health concerns, receive medical advice, and even obtain prescriptions without ever leaving their home. This ease of access not only saves time and effort but also encourages regular check-ins and follow-ups, leading to better overall health outcomes.

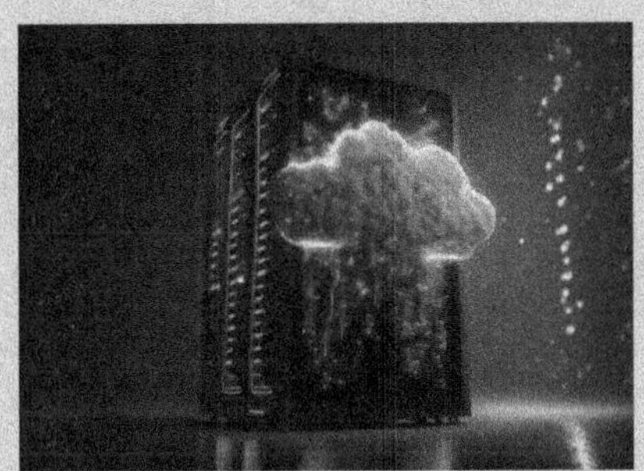

Those living in remote areas with limited access to healthcare facilities can greatly benefit from telemedicine consultations. By connecting with doctors and specialists remotely, individuals in underserved communities can access the same level of care as those in urban areas. This can be especially crucial for managing chronic conditions or seeking specialized medical advice, ensuring that everyone has equal access to quality healthcare regardless of their location.

Cost-conscious individuals will also appreciate the potential for lower healthcare costs with telemedicine. By avoiding the expenses associated with in-person visits, such as transportation and childcare, patients can save money while still receiving the same level of care. Additionally, telemedicine can help prevent unnecessary emergency room visits by providing timely consultations and monitoring, ultimately reducing overall healthcare spending for both patients and providers.

For parents of young children, individuals with chronic conditions, and the elderly, telemedicine offers a convenient and accessible option for healthcare consultations. From minor illnesses to chronic disease management, telemedicine can provide regular follow-up appointments, specialist consultations, and monitoring, all from the comfort of home. This not only saves time and effort but also ensures that healthcare remains a priority for all individuals, regardless of their age or health status.

Prescriptions and Referrals through Telemedicine

Telemedicine is revolutionizing the way healthcare is delivered, making it easier than ever for busy professionals to access medical consultations without having to take time off work. With telemedicine, individuals can schedule appointments at their convenience, eliminating the need to sit in a crowded waiting room for hours. This flexibility is especially beneficial for those with demanding schedules who struggle to find time for traditional in-person doctor visits.

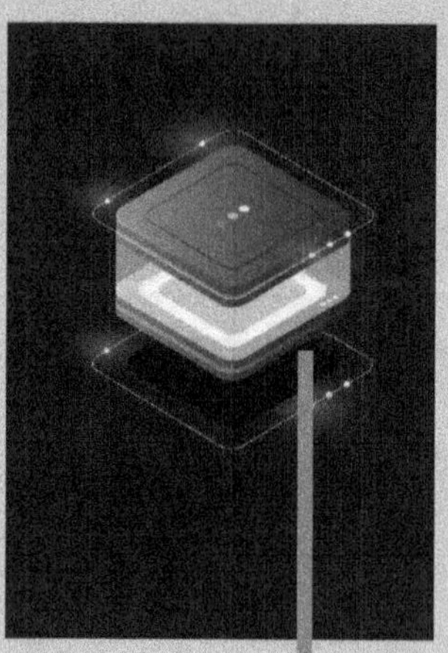

Telemedicine Revolution: How to Take Control of Your Health Anytime, Anywhere

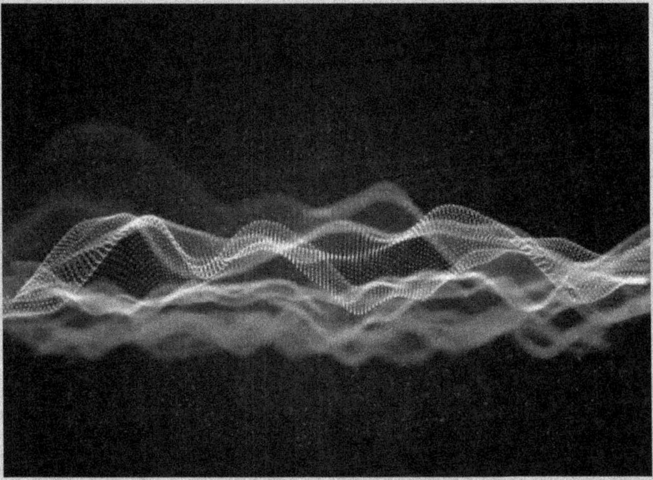

Tech savvy individuals will appreciate the ease and convenience of telemedicine consultations. With just a click of a button, patients can connect with a healthcare provider from the comfort of their own home. Prescriptions and referrals can be easily obtained through telemedicine, allowing individuals to receive the care they need without the hassle of scheduling an in-person appointment.

For those living in remote areas with limited access to healthcare facilities, telemedicine can be a lifesaver. Telemedicine consultations can bridge the gap between patients and healthcare providers, ensuring that individuals in rural or underserved communities have access to quality care. Prescriptions and referrals can be easily obtained through telemedicine, providing essential medical services to those who may not have easy access to traditional healthcare facilities.

Cost conscious individuals will appreciate the potential cost savings associated with telemedicine. By opting for remote consultations instead of traditional in-person visits, patients can avoid costly co-pays and transportation expenses. Telemedicine can be a cost-effective solution for those looking to manage their healthcare expenses while still receiving quality medical care.

In conclusion telemedicine offers a convenient and accessible option for obtaining prescriptions and referrals from healthcare providers Whether you are a busy professional a tech savvy individual or someone living in a remote area telemedicine can provide you with the care you need without the hassle of traditional in person visits By taking advantage of telemedicine you can take control of your health anytime anywhere

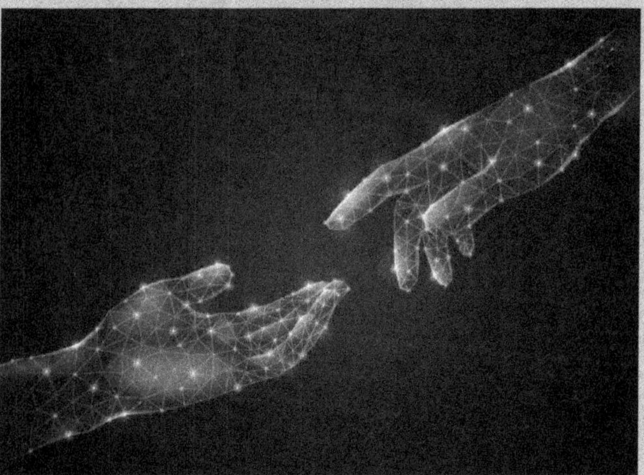

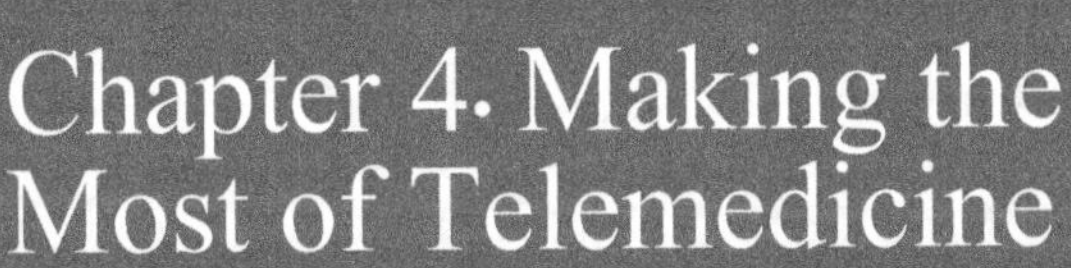

Chapter 4. Making the Most of Telemedicine

Choosing a Telemedicine Provider

Choosing a telemedicine provider can be a daunting task, especially with the growing number of options available in the market. When selecting a telemedicine provider, it is essential to consider the specific needs and preferences of the individual. For busy professionals who struggle to find time for traditional doctor appointments, a telemedicine provider that offers flexible scheduling and quick consultations may be the best fit. Tech-savvy individuals may prefer a provider that offers a user-friendly platform and a seamless digital experience. For those living in remote areas with limited access to healthcare facilities, it is crucial to choose a telemedicine provider that offers a wide network of healthcare professionals and specialists. Cost-conscious individuals should look for providers that offer affordable pricing options and transparent fee structures. It is important to research and compare different telemedicine providers to find one that aligns with your budget and healthcare needs. Parents of young children can benefit from telemedicine providers that offer pediatric services and virtual consultations for minor illnesses or routine checkups. Individuals managing chronic conditions may require specialized care and regular follow-up appointments with healthcare professionals. It is important to choose a telemedicine provider that offers access to specialists in your specific medical condition.

For the elderly population telemedicine can provide easier access to healthcare services without the need for extensive travel. It is essential to choose a telemedicine provider that offers support for older adults including easy to use technology and personalized care options. Ultimately selecting the right telemedicine provider is crucial for taking control of your health and accessing quality healthcare services anytime anywhere

Preparing for a Telemedicine Consultation

Preparing for a telemedicine consultation can be a simple and stress free process especially for busy professionals who struggle to find time for in person doctor appointments. The first step is to ensure you have a stable internet connection and a device with a camera such as a smartphone tablet or computer. This will allow you to easily connect with your healthcare provider from anywhere whether it be your office home or even while traveling

Tech-savvy individuals will appreciate the convenience and ease of telemedicine consultations. Familiarize yourself with the telemedicine platform or app that your healthcare provider uses before your appointment. This will help you feel more comfortable navigating the virtual visit and ensure a smooth experience. Be sure to test your camera and microphone beforehand to ensure they are working properly.

For those living in remote areas with limited access to healthcare facilities, telemedicine consultations can be a game-changer. Make sure to gather any relevant medical records or information before your appointment. This will help your healthcare provider make an accurate assessment and provide the best possible care. Be prepared to discuss your symptoms, medical history, and any medications you are currently taking during the consultation.

Cost-conscious individuals will appreciate the potential cost savings of telemedicine compared to traditional in-person visits. Check with your insurance provider to see if telemedicine consultations are covered under your plan. Some providers may offer telemedicine services at a lower cost than in-person visits, making it a more affordable option for routine medical care.

Overall, preparing for a telemedicine consultation is a simple process that can benefit a wide range of individuals. Whether you are a busy professional, tech-savvy individual, or live in a remote area, telemedicine offers a flexible and convenient solution for accessing healthcare. By following these tips and being prepared for your appointment, you can take control of your health anytime, anywhere.

Understanding Telemedicine Etiquette

In today's fast-paced world, telemedicine has become a popular and convenient option for individuals looking to take control of their health without having to disrupt their busy schedules. Whether you are a busy professional, tech-savvy individual, or someone living in a remote location with limited access to healthcare facilities, telemedicine offers a flexible solution for consultations. However, just like any other form of communication, there are certain etiquette guidelines that should be followed to ensure a successful and productive telemedicine visit.

First and foremost, it is important to treat a telemedicine consultation with the same level of professionalism and respect as an in-person doctor visit. This means being on time for your appointment, dressing appropriately, and finding a quiet and private space to conduct the call. Remember, your doctor is still providing you with valuable medical advice and deserves your full attention and respect.

Secondly, communication is key in a telemedicine consultation. Be prepared to clearly and concisely explain your symptoms, medical history, and any medications you may be taking. It is also important to actively listen to your doctor's recommendations and ask any questions you may have. Remember, the more information you provide, the better your doctor will be able to help you.

Additionally, it is important to remember that telemedicine is not a replacement for emergency medical care. If you are experiencing a life-threatening emergency, you should seek immediate medical attention at the nearest hospital or emergency room. Telemedicine is best suited for non-emergency medical issues such as minor illnesses, follow-up appointments, or routine checkups.

Furthermore, be mindful of the technology you are using for your telemedicine consultation. Make sure that your internet connection is stable and that your camera and microphone are working properly. If you are not familiar with the telemedicine platform being used, take some time to familiarize yourself with it before your appointment to avoid any technical difficulties.

In conclusion, understanding and following telemedicine etiquette is essential for a successful and productive remote doctor visit. By treating the consultation with professionalism, communicating effectively, and being mindful of the technology being used, you can make the most out of your telemedicine experience. Embracing telemedicine as a convenient and cost-effective option for healthcare can lead to better health outcomes and more efficient use of your time.

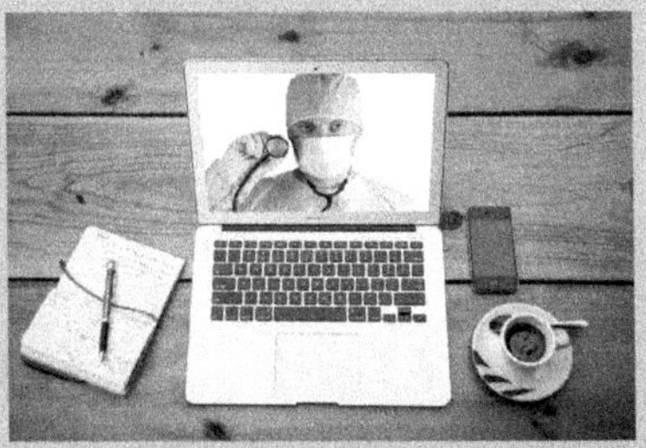

Ensuring Privacy and Security in Telemedicine

In a world where time is of the essence and convenience is key, telemedicine has emerged as a revolutionary solution for individuals seeking healthcare services without the hassle of traditional in-person visits. Ensuring privacy and security in telemedicine is paramount to provide a safe and reliable platform for consultations. Busy professionals, tech-savvy individuals, those living in remote areas, and cost-conscious people can all benefit from the convenience of telemedicine consultations. By addressing the needs of these primary audiences, telemedicine can truly revolutionize the way healthcare is accessed and delivered.

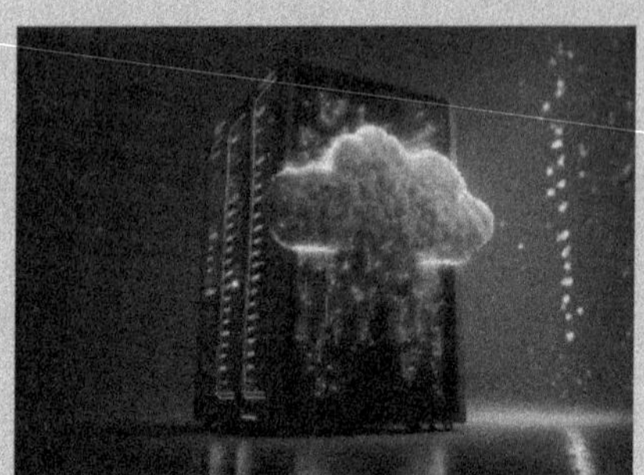

One of the key considerations in telemedicine is the protection of patient information and maintaining the highest standards of privacy and security. It is essential for telemedicine platforms to use secure and encrypted communication channels to ensure that patient data remains confidential. Providers should also adhere to strict privacy protocols and comply with regulations such as HIPAA to safeguard patient information. By prioritizing privacy and security in telemedicine, individuals can feel confident in the safety of their consultations and medical records.

For busy professionals with demanding schedules, telemedicine offers a flexible solution for accessing healthcare services without having to take time off work for doctor appointments. By being able to consult with healthcare providers remotely, busy professionals can receive the care they need without disrupting their work commitments. Tech savvy individuals who are comfortable using technology will appreciate the ease and convenience of remote doctor visits, allowing them to take control of their health anytime, anywhere.

Individuals living in remote areas with limited access to healthcare facilities can benefit greatly from telemedicine consultations. By providing a virtual platform for medical appointments, telemedicine bridges the gap between patients and healthcare providers, ensuring that individuals in underserved areas have access to quality healthcare services. Additionally, for cost conscious people looking to reduce healthcare expenses, telemedicine can potentially lead to lower costs compared to traditional in person visits, making healthcare more affordable and accessible for all.

By addressing the needs of primary audiences such as busy professionals, tech savvy individuals, those living in remote areas, and cost conscious people, telemedicine can truly revolutionize the way healthcare is accessed and delivered. By ensuring privacy and security in telemedicine, individuals can feel confident in the safety of their consultations and medical records. With the convenience of telemedicine, individuals can take charge of their health anytime, anywhere, without the constraints of traditional in person visits.

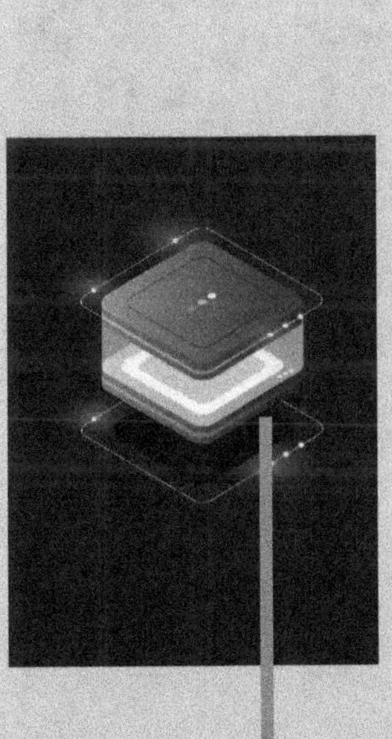

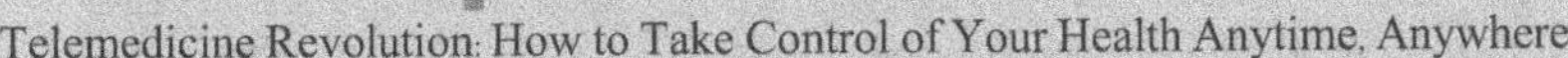

Telemedicine Revolution: How to Take Control of Your Health Anytime, Anywhere

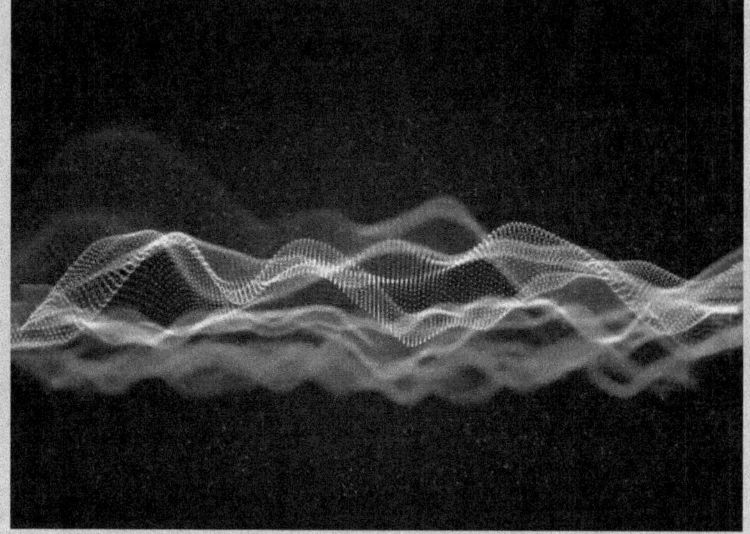

Telemedicine Revolution: How to Take Control of Your Health Anytime, Anywhere

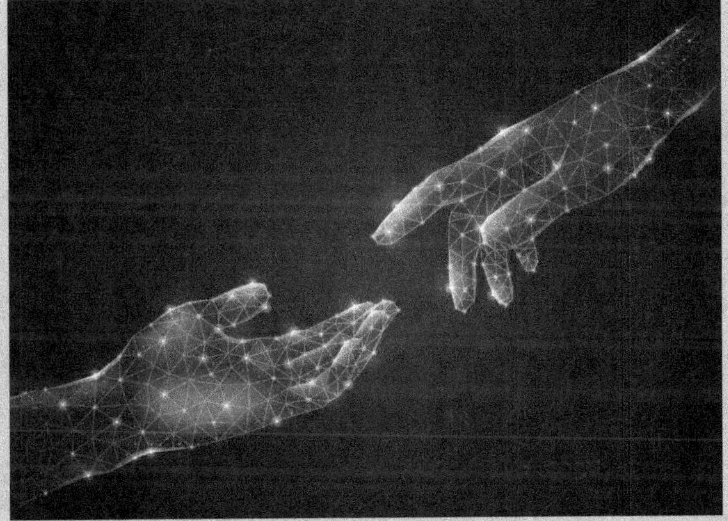

Chapter 5: Telemedicine for Busy Professionals

Benefits of Telemedicine for Busy Professionals

In today's fast-paced world, busy professionals often find it challenging to prioritize their health amidst their demanding schedules. However, with the advent of telemedicine, individuals can now access healthcare services without having to take time off work for traditional in-person doctor appointments. This flexible solution allows professionals to schedule consultations at their convenience, whether it be during their lunch break or after work hours. By utilizing telemedicine, busy professionals can take control of their health anytime, anywhere.

For tech-savvy individuals who are comfortable using technology, telemedicine offers a seamless and convenient way to connect with healthcare providers. With just a few clicks, individuals can easily access virtual consultations with doctors, specialists, or therapists. This eliminates the need for lengthy commutes and waiting room delays, making it a time-efficient option for those who value convenience and efficiency in their healthcare experience.

Individuals living in remote areas with limited access to healthcare facilities can greatly benefit from telemedicine consultations. By leveraging technology, these locationally challenged individuals can receive quality healthcare services without the need to travel long distances. Telemedicine bridges the gap between healthcare providers and patients, ensuring that everyone has access to medical expertise regardless of their geographical location.

One of the key advantages of telemedicine is its potential to lower healthcare costs compared to traditional in person visits. By eliminating the need for travel expenses and reducing the overhead costs associated with physical clinics, telemedicine can offer cost conscious individuals a more affordable option for consultations. This can be particularly beneficial for those who require frequent follow up appointments or routine check ups.

In conclusion, telemedicine is a game changer for busy professionals and individuals in various niches who face challenges in accessing traditional healthcare services. Whether you are a tech savvy individual, someone living in a remote area, or a cost conscious individual, telemedicine offers a flexible, convenient, and cost effective solution for taking control of your health. By embracing the telemedicine revolution, you can prioritize your well being without compromising your busy schedule.

Managing Health on a Tight Schedule

In today's fast-paced world, managing your health can often feel like just another task on your never-ending to-do list. For busy professionals, finding the time to schedule and attend doctor appointments can be a challenge. Telemedicine offers a flexible solution for consultations, allowing you to take control of your health on your own terms. By utilizing telemedicine, you can easily fit in appointments during your lunch break or after work, without having to take time off or rearrange your schedule. For tech-savvy individuals, the convenience of remote doctor visits is a game-changer. With just a few clicks on your smartphone or computer, you can connect with healthcare professionals and receive the care you need. Telemedicine platforms are designed to be user-friendly and intuitive, making it easy for anyone comfortable using technology to navigate the virtual healthcare landscape. Whether you're seeking advice on minor ailments or follow-up care for chronic conditions, telemedicine puts the power of healthcare in your hands.

Living in a remote area with limited access to healthcare facilities can present a unique set of challenges when it comes to managing your health. Telemedicine consultations bridge the gap between patients and providers, offering a convenient way to receive medical advice and treatment without the need for long commutes or expensive travel. Whether you're miles away from the nearest medical facility or simply prefer the convenience of virtual visits, telemedicine can be a lifesaver for those who are locationally challenged.

For cost-conscious individuals, telemedicine offers the potential for lower healthcare costs compared to traditional in-person visits. By eliminating travel expenses and reducing the need for office visits, telemedicine can help you save money while still receiving high-quality care. With affordable subscription plans and pay-as-you-go options, telemedicine makes it easy to prioritize your health without breaking the bank.

In conclusion, telemedicine is revolutionizing the way we approach healthcare, offering a convenient and cost-effective solution for managing your health on a tight schedule. Whether you're a busy professional, a tech-savvy individual, or someone living in a remote area, telemedicine can provide the care you need when you need it. By taking advantage of telemedicine services, you can ditch the waiting room and take charge of your health from anywhere. Remember, your health is your greatest asset — make it a priority, no matter how busy life gets.

Integrating Telemedicine into Work Life

Integrating telemedicine into work life can revolutionize the way busy professionals manage their health. With demanding schedules and limited time off, it can be challenging to fit in traditional doctor appointments. Telemedicine offers a flexible solution that allows individuals to consult with healthcare providers from the convenience of their workplace or home. By utilizing telemedicine, busy professionals can prioritize their health without sacrificing productivity. Tech savvy individuals will appreciate the ease and convenience of telemedicine consultations. With just a few clicks, they can connect with a healthcare provider and receive the care they need without the hassle of scheduling appointments or commuting to a physical office. Telemedicine harnesses the power of technology to make healthcare more accessible and convenient for those comfortable with digital platforms.

For those living in remote areas with limited access to healthcare facilities, telemedicine can be a lifeline. By connecting with healthcare providers through telemedicine platforms, individuals in locationally challenged areas can receive quality care without the need to travel long distances. Telemedicine bridges the gap between patients and providers, ensuring that everyone has access to the healthcare they need, regardless of their geographic location. Cost conscious individuals will appreciate the potential cost savings that telemedicine can offer. By eliminating the need for travel and reducing overhead costs associated with in person visits, telemedicine consultations can be a more affordable option for managing health concerns. With telemedicine, individuals can prioritize their health without breaking the bank, making it a cost effective solution for those looking to save money on healthcare expenses.

In conclusion, integrating telemedicine into work life can benefit a wide range of individuals, from busy professionals to the elderly. By embracing telemedicine as a convenient and accessible option for healthcare consultations, individuals can take control of their health anytime, anywhere. Whether you are a tech-savvy individual, a cost-conscious person, or someone living in a remote area, telemedicine offers a solution that can revolutionize the way you manage your health.

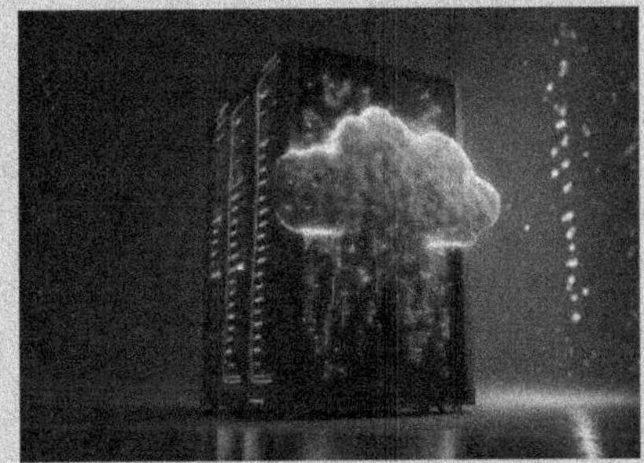

Maximizing Productivity with Telemedicine

Maximizing productivity with telemedicine is a game-changer for busy professionals who struggle to find time for traditional doctor appointments. With telemedicine, individuals can schedule consultations around their demanding work schedules, eliminating the need to take time off or rearrange their day. This flexibility allows for seamless integration of healthcare into their busy lives, ultimately leading to increased productivity and peace of mind.

For tech-savvy individuals, telemedicine offers the convenience of remote consultations at the touch of a button. With the rise of mobile health apps and virtual platforms, accessing healthcare has never been easier. Whether it's a quick check-in with a doctor or a follow-up appointment with a specialist, telemedicine provides a hassle-free solution for those comfortable with using technology to manage their health.

Those living in remote areas with limited access to healthcare facilities can greatly benefit from telemedicine consultations. By connecting with healthcare providers virtually, individuals can receive quality medical care without the need to travel long distances. This accessibility not only saves time and money but also ensures that individuals in underserved areas have equal access to healthcare services.

Cost conscious individuals can also take advantage of telemedicine to potentially lower their healthcare expenses. With telemedicine consultations typically costing less than traditional in person visits, individuals can save money on co pays, transportation, and time away from work. By maximizing the efficiency of telemedicine, individuals can prioritize their health without breaking the bank.

In addition to busy professionals, tech savvy individuals, and those living in remote areas, telemedicine also serves as a convenient option for parents of young children, individuals with chronic conditions, and the elderly. By offering easier access to healthcare and eliminating barriers to traditional appointments, telemedicine empowers individuals to take control of their health from anywhere. By embracing the telemedicine revolution, individuals can ditch the waiting room and embrace a new era of healthcare that puts their needs first.

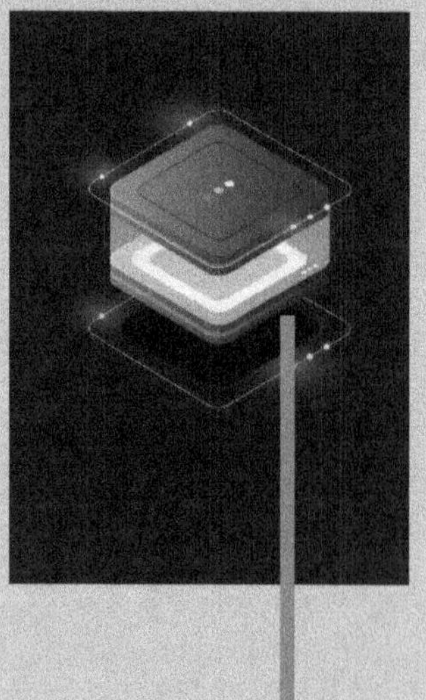

Telemedicine Revolution: How to Take Control of Your Health Anytime, Anywhere

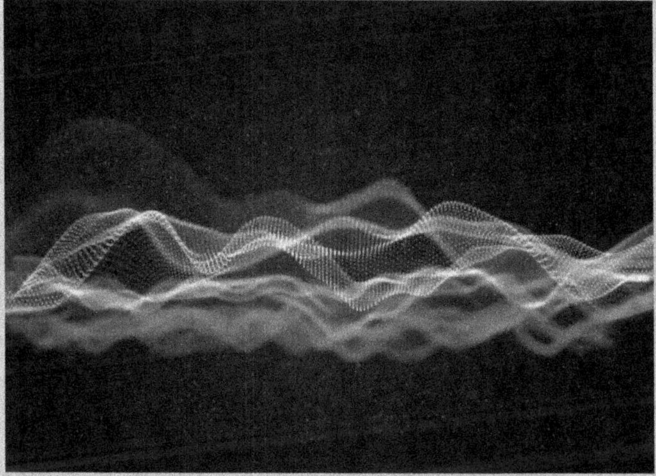

Chapter 6: Telemedicine for Tech-Savvy Individuals

Embracing Technology in Healthcare

In today's fast-paced world, it can be challenging for busy professionals to find the time to schedule and attend doctor appointments. This is where telemedicine comes in, offering a flexible solution for consultations that can be done anytime, anywhere. With the ability to connect with healthcare providers remotely, busy professionals can take control of their health without having to take time off work or rearrange their schedules.

For tech-savvy individuals who are comfortable using technology, telemedicine offers the ease and convenience of remote doctor visits. With just a few clicks, you can connect with a healthcare provider and receive the care you need without having to leave the comfort of your home. This modern approach to healthcare is perfect for those who value convenience and efficiency in their busy lives.

Living in remote areas with limited access to healthcare facilities can make it difficult to receive the medical attention you need. Telemedicine consultations can bridge this gap, offering locationally challenged individuals the opportunity to connect with healthcare providers without having to travel long distances. This can be especially beneficial for those who live in rural areas and may not have easy access to traditional in-person doctor visits.

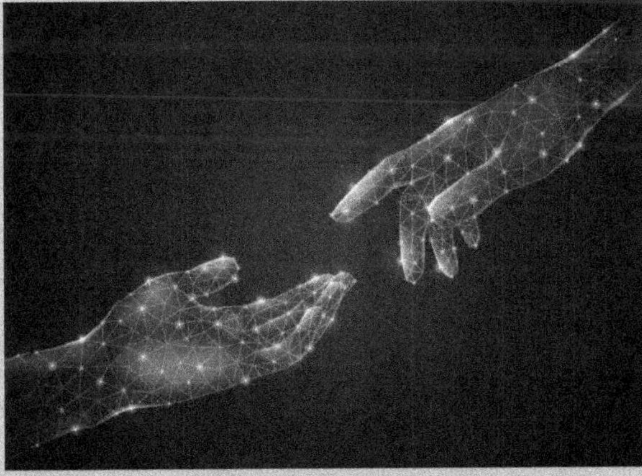

For cost-conscious individuals, telemedicine can potentially lead to lower healthcare costs compared to traditional in-person visits. By avoiding travel expenses and reducing the need for time off work, telemedicine consultations can be a more affordable option for those looking to save money on their healthcare expenses. This cost-effective approach to healthcare can help individuals take charge of their health without breaking the bank.

In conclusion, telemedicine is a revolutionary way to embrace technology in healthcare and take control of your health anytime, anywhere. Whether you are a busy professional, a tech-savvy individual, locationally challenged, or cost-conscious, telemedicine offers a convenient and efficient solution for your healthcare needs. By ditching the waiting room and opting for telemedicine consultations, you can prioritize your health and well-being without sacrificing your busy lifestyle.

Navigating Telemedicine Platforms

In today's fast-paced world, finding time to visit the doctor can be a challenge for many busy professionals. Telemedicine offers a flexible solution for consultations that can be done anytime, anywhere. With just a few clicks on your smartphone or computer, you can connect with a healthcare provider and receive the care you need without having to take time off work. This convenience makes telemedicine a popular choice for individuals with demanding schedules who value their time.

For tech savvy individuals who are comfortable using technology, telemedicine platforms offer an easy and convenient way to access healthcare services. With user friendly interfaces and secure communication channels, these platforms make it simple to schedule appointments, upload medical records, and communicate with healthcare providers. The ability to have remote doctor visits from the comfort of your own home or office appeals to those who appreciate the efficiency and convenience that telemedicine offers.

Living in remote areas with limited access to healthcare facilities can present challenges when seeking medical care. Telemedicine consultations bridge the gap for locationally challenged individuals by providing access to healthcare services no matter where they are located. Whether you are miles away from the nearest clinic or simply prefer the convenience of virtual visits, telemedicine platforms offer a lifeline for those who face barriers to traditional in person appointments.

For cost-conscious individuals looking to save money on healthcare expenses, telemedicine can be a cost-effective alternative to traditional in-person visits. By eliminating the need for travel expenses, parking fees, and other associated costs, telemedicine consultations can potentially lead to lower healthcare expenses overall. This financial benefit makes telemedicine an attractive option for those who want to take control of their health without breaking the bank.

In conclusion, navigating telemedicine platforms is a valuable skill for a variety of audiences, including busy professionals, tech-savvy individuals, those living in remote areas, and cost-conscious individuals. By taking advantage of the convenience, accessibility, and cost-saving benefits of telemedicine, individuals can take control of their health anytime, anywhere. Whether you are a parent of young children, managing chronic conditions, or an older adult seeking easier access to healthcare, telemedicine platforms offer a solution that fits your needs and lifestyle.

Leveraging Health Apps and Wearables

In today's fast-paced world, it can be challenging to find the time to schedule and attend in-person doctor appointments. For busy professionals who are constantly on the go, telemedicine offers a flexible solution that allows them to consult with healthcare providers from anywhere, at any time. By leveraging health apps and wearables, individuals can easily monitor their health and communicate with medical professionals without disrupting their demanding schedules.

Tech-savvy individuals who are comfortable using technology will appreciate the ease and convenience of remote doctor visits. With the rise of telemedicine platforms and mobile health apps, accessing healthcare services has never been easier. By utilizing wearable devices that track vital signs and health data, individuals can provide their healthcare providers with valuable information that can aid in diagnosis and treatment.

For those living in remote areas with limited access to healthcare facilities, telemedicine consultations can be a lifesaver. By leveraging telemedicine technology, individuals in rural or underserved areas can connect with healthcare providers and specialists without the need to travel long distances. This not only saves time and money but also ensures that individuals receive the care they need in a timely manner.

Cost-conscious individuals can also benefit from telemedicine, as it has the potential to lower healthcare costs compared to traditional, in-person visits. By reducing the need for unnecessary office visits and travel expenses, telemedicine can help individuals save money while still receiving quality healthcare services. Additionally, telemedicine consultations are often covered by insurance, making it an affordable option for those looking to take control of their health.

For parents of young children, individuals with chronic conditions, and the elderly, telemedicine offers a convenient and accessible option for healthcare consultations. Whether it's a minor illness, a regular follow-up appointment, or difficulty traveling to in-person visits, telemedicine can provide a solution for individuals of all ages and backgrounds. By leveraging health apps and wearables, individuals can take charge of their health from anywhere and ensure that they receive the care they need, when they need it.

Staying Connected with Telehealth Providers

In today's fast-paced world, staying connected with healthcare providers can be a challenge for many individuals, especially those with demanding schedules. For busy professionals who find it difficult to take time off work for doctor appointments, telemedicine offers a flexible solution. With the ability to schedule remote consultations at a time that works best for you, telemedicine allows you to take control of your health anytime, anywhere.

Tech-savvy individuals will appreciate the ease and convenience of telemedicine. With just a few clicks on your smartphone or computer, you can connect with a healthcare provider for a virtual visit. Gone are the days of waiting in crowded waiting rooms or trying to schedule appointments around your busy day. Telemedicine puts the power of healthcare in the palm of your hand.

For those living in remote areas with limited access to healthcare facilities, telemedicine consultations can be a lifesaver. Whether you're miles away from the nearest doctor's office or simply don't have the means to travel for an appointment, telemedicine offers a convenient solution. By staying connected with telehealth providers, you can receive the care you need without the hassle of long commutes or expensive travel costs.

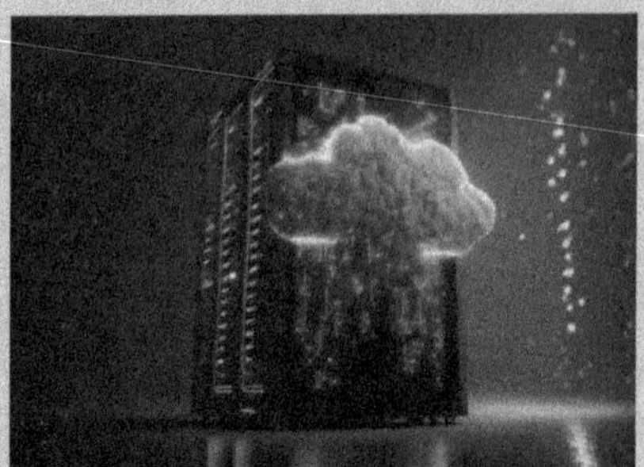

Cost-conscious individuals will also find telemedicine to be a valuable resource. With the potential for lower healthcare costs compared to traditional in-person visits, telemedicine can help you save money while still receiving quality care. Whether you're seeking treatment for a minor illness or need a follow-up consultation with a specialist, telemedicine offers an affordable alternative to traditional healthcare services.

For parents of young children, individuals with chronic conditions, and the elderly, telemedicine can offer easier access to healthcare. Whether you're seeking a consultation for a minor illness in your child, managing a chronic condition with regular follow-up appointments, or need easier access to healthcare as an older adult, telemedicine can help you take charge of your health from anywhere. By staying connected with telehealth providers, you can receive the care you need without the inconvenience of traditional in-person visits.

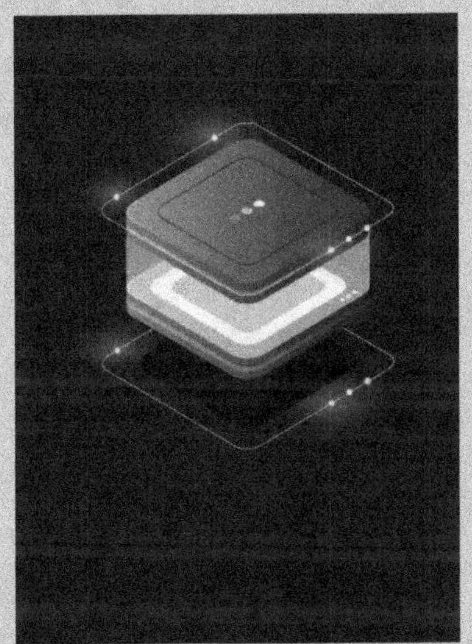

Telemedicine Revolution: How to Take Control of Your Health Anytime, Anywhere

Chapter 7: Telemedicine for Locationally Challenged Individuals

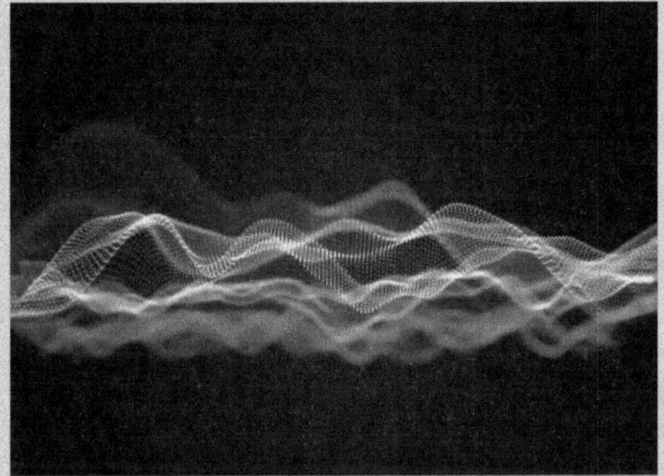

Overcoming Healthcare Barriers with Telemedicine

In today's fast-paced world, many individuals, especially busy professionals, find it challenging to take time off work for traditional doctor appointments. This is where telemedicine comes in as a game-changer, offering a flexible solution for consultations. With telemedicine, individuals can schedule appointments at their convenience, without having to worry about commuting to a physical healthcare facility. This not only saves time but also provides the opportunity for individuals to prioritize their health without sacrificing their work commitments.

For tech-savvy individuals who are comfortable using technology, telemedicine offers the ease and convenience of remote doctor visits. Through video calls, phone consultations, and secure messaging platforms, individuals can connect with healthcare providers from anywhere, using their smartphones or computers. This accessibility not only streamlines the healthcare process but also empowers individuals to take control of their health in a way that fits their tech-savvy lifestyle.

Individuals living in remote areas with limited access to healthcare facilities often face challenges when it comes to receiving timely medical care. Telemedicine bridges this gap by allowing individuals to consult with healthcare providers remotely. This is especially beneficial for those who may not have easy access to specialists or healthcare services in their area. By overcoming location barriers, telemedicine ensures that everyone has equal access to quality healthcare, regardless of where they live.

For cost-conscious individuals, telemedicine can potentially lead to lower healthcare costs compared to traditional in-person visits. With telemedicine, individuals can save money on transportation, parking, and time off work, as well as avoid unnecessary emergency room visits for non-emergency issues. By utilizing telemedicine services, individuals can reduce their healthcare expenses while still receiving high-quality medical care from the comfort of their own home.

For parents of young children, individuals with chronic conditions, and the elderly, telemedicine offers a convenient and accessible option for healthcare consultations. Whether it's for minor illnesses, regular follow-up appointments, or managing chronic conditions, telemedicine provides a way for individuals to stay connected with healthcare providers without the hassle of traveling to a physical office. By embracing telemedicine, individuals can take charge of their health from anywhere, ensuring that they receive the care they need, when they need it.

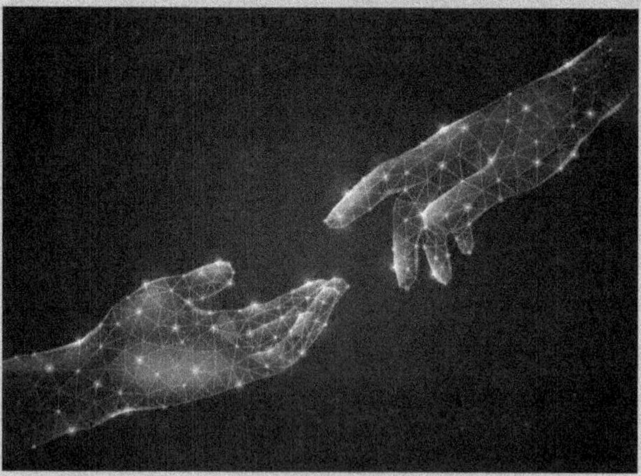

Accessing Specialists through Telemedicine

Busy professionals, tech savvy individuals, those living in remote areas, and cost conscious people can all benefit from accessing specialists through telemedicine. With demanding schedules, it can be difficult for busy professionals to take time off work for doctor appointments. Telemedicine offers a flexible solution, allowing them to have consultations with specialists at their convenience. For tech savvy individuals who are comfortable using technology, remote doctor visits provide ease and convenience without the hassle of traveling to a physical office.

Individuals living in remote areas with limited access to healthcare facilities can greatly benefit from telemedicine consultations. Telemedicine bridges the gap between patients and specialists, providing access to quality healthcare regardless of location. Additionally, for those who are cost conscious, telemedicine can potentially lead to lower healthcare costs compared to traditional in person visits. By eliminating the need for travel and reducing overhead costs, telemedicine offers a more affordable option for accessing specialist care.

For parents of young children, telemedicine can be a convenient option for consultations regarding minor illnesses or checkups. Instead of taking time off work and traveling to a doctor's office, parents can easily connect with specialists through telemedicine for quick and efficient consultations. Individuals managing chronic conditions may also benefit from regular telemedicine follow-up appointments with specialists. Telemedicine provides a convenient way to monitor and manage chronic conditions without the need for frequent in-person visits.

For the elderly, telemedicine offers easier access to healthcare without the hassle of traveling for appointments. Older adults who may have difficulty getting to a doctor's office can benefit from telemedicine consultations with specialists from the comfort of their own home. Telemedicine revolutionizes the way healthcare is accessed and provides a convenient and cost-effective solution for individuals of all ages and backgrounds. By taking advantage of telemedicine, individuals can take control of their health anytime, anywhere, without the constraints of traditional healthcare systems.

Improving Healthcare Equity with Telehealth

Healthcare equity is a pressing issue that affects millions of people around the world. One solution that has gained traction in recent years is telehealth, a revolutionary approach that allows individuals to connect with healthcare providers remotely. This innovative technology is particularly valuable for busy professionals who struggle to find time for in-person doctor appointments. With telemedicine, consultations can be scheduled at a time that works best for the patient, eliminating the need to take time off work or rearrange schedules.

For tech-savvy individuals, telehealth offers a convenient and easy-to-use platform for accessing healthcare services. By simply logging onto a secure online portal, patients can connect with their healthcare providers for consultations, follow-ups, and even prescriptions. The ease and convenience of telemedicine make it an attractive option for those who are comfortable using technology to manage their health.

Another group that can benefit greatly from telehealth services are individuals who live in remote or underserved areas with limited access to healthcare facilities. For these locationally challenged individuals, telemedicine consultations can bridge the gap between them and quality healthcare services. By connecting with healthcare providers remotely, patients can receive the care they need without having to travel long distances or incur significant costs.

In addition to improving access to healthcare, telemedicine also has the potential to lower healthcare costs for patients. By reducing the need for in-person visits, telehealth can help cut down on transportation expenses, time off work, and other associated costs. This makes telemedicine an attractive option for cost-conscious individuals who are looking for ways to save money on healthcare services.

For parents of young children, individuals with chronic conditions, and the elderly, telemedicine offers a convenient and accessible way to manage their health. Whether it's scheduling regular check-ups for children, follow-up appointments for chronic conditions, or consultations for elderly adults who have difficulty traveling, telehealth can provide a valuable solution for individuals in these demographics. By embracing telemedicine, individuals can take control of their health from anywhere, at any time.

Telemedicine for Rural and Underserved Communities

Telemedicine has become a game-changer for rural and underserved communities, providing a much-needed solution for individuals who struggle to access traditional healthcare services. For our primary audience of busy professionals, telemedicine offers a flexible alternative to in-person doctor appointments. With the ability to schedule consultations around their demanding schedules, busy professionals can take control of their health without having to take time off work.

Tech-savvy individuals will also appreciate the convenience of telemedicine, as they are comfortable using technology to connect with healthcare providers remotely. This allows them to access medical advice and support anytime, anywhere, without the need to physically visit a doctor's office. For those who are locationally challenged, such as those living in remote areas with limited access to healthcare facilities, telemedicine can bridge the gap and provide much-needed medical consultations.

Cost-conscious individuals will also benefit from telemedicine, as it can potentially lead to lower healthcare costs compared to traditional in-person visits. By eliminating the need for travel expenses and reducing wait times, telemedicine offers a cost-effective option for those looking to save money on healthcare services. In addition, our secondary audience of parents of young children can take advantage of telemedicine for minor illnesses or checkups, saving them time and hassle.

For individuals with chronic conditions, telemedicine offers a convenient way to stay in touch with specialists and receive regular follow-up care. This can help them better manage their conditions and stay on top of their health without the need for frequent in-person visits. Lastly, telemedicine can provide easier access to healthcare for the elderly, who may have difficulty traveling for appointments. By offering remote consultations, older adults can receive the care they need without the added stress of transportation and waiting rooms. Overall, telemedicine is revolutionizing the way healthcare is delivered, making it easier and more convenient for all individuals to take control of their health from anywhere.

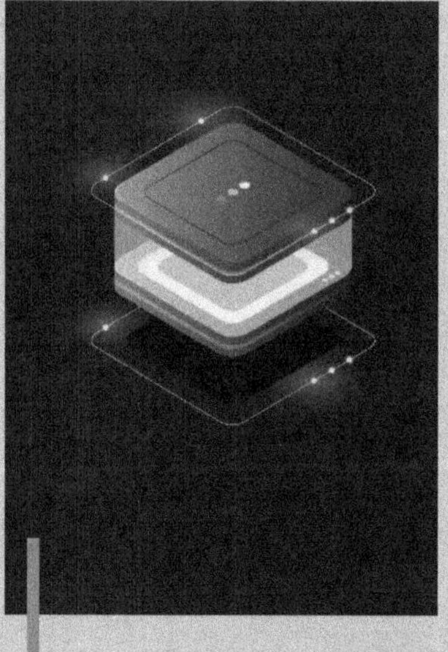

Telemedicine Revolution: How to Take Control of Your Health Anytime, Anywhere

Chapter 8: Telemedicine for Cost-Conscious Consumers

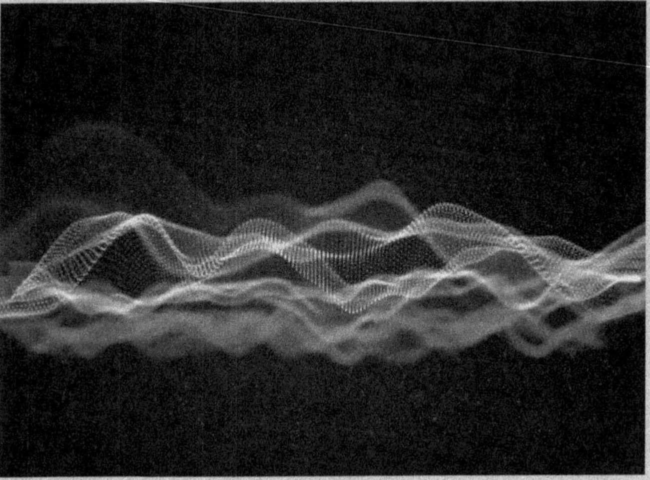

Saving Money with Telemedicine

Saving money with telemedicine is a key benefit that many busy professionals, tech-savvy individuals, locationally challenged individuals, and cost-conscious people can take advantage of. With telemedicine, you can easily consult with a healthcare provider without having to take time off work for in-person appointments. This flexibility allows you to prioritize your health without sacrificing your professional commitments.

For busy professionals, telemedicine offers a convenient solution to fit healthcare appointments into their demanding schedules. By eliminating the need to travel to a doctor's office and wait in a waiting room, telemedicine saves time and allows professionals to focus on their work while still receiving necessary medical care.

Tech-savvy individuals will appreciate the ease and convenience of remote doctor visits through telemedicine. With just a few clicks on a computer or smartphone, you can connect with a healthcare provider for a virtual consultation. This streamlined process not only saves time but also reduces the hassle of scheduling and traveling to appointments.

People living in remote areas with limited access to healthcare facilities can benefit significantly from telemedicine consultations. By leveraging technology to connect with healthcare providers, individuals in rural or underserved areas can access quality medical care without the need to travel long distances, saving both time and money.

Cost conscious individuals will find that telemedicine can potentially lead to lower healthcare costs compared to traditional in person visits. With telemedicine, you can avoid additional expenses such as transportation costs, parking fees, and missed work hours. By opting for telemedicine consultations, you can take control of your health while also saving money in the process.

Comparing Telemedicine Costs to Traditional Healthcare

Telemedicine has emerged as a cost effective alternative to traditional healthcare, offering numerous benefits to individuals across various demographics. Busy professionals, in particular, can benefit from the flexibility of telemedicine consultations, as they can easily fit appointments into their demanding schedules without the need to take time off work. This convenience can lead to increased productivity and reduced stress for those juggling multiple responsibilities.

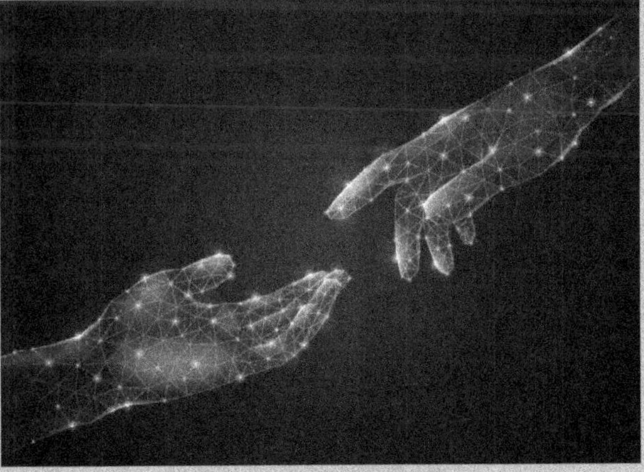

For tech-savvy individuals, telemedicine provides a streamlined and convenient way to access healthcare services. With the click of a button, individuals can connect with healthcare professionals from the comfort of their own homes, saving time and eliminating the need for travel to a physical office. This accessibility is especially appealing to those who are comfortable using technology and prefer the convenience of remote consultations.

Individuals living in remote areas with limited access to healthcare facilities can greatly benefit from telemedicine services. By eliminating the need for long travel distances to see a doctor, telemedicine offers a practical solution for those who may otherwise struggle to receive timely medical care. This increased accessibility can lead to improved health outcomes for individuals in underserved communities.

In terms of cost-conscious individuals, telemedicine can potentially lead to lower healthcare costs compared to traditional in-person visits. With reduced overhead expenses and the ability to see patients more efficiently, healthcare providers offering telemedicine services can pass on these cost savings to their patients. This cost effectiveness makes telemedicine an attractive option for those looking to save money on healthcare expenses.

Telemedicine Revolution: How to Take Control of Your Health Anytime, Anywhere

Overall, telemedicine offers a convenient and cost-effective healthcare solution for a wide range of individuals, including busy professionals, tech-savvy individuals, and those living in remote areas. By leveraging technology to connect patients with healthcare professionals, telemedicine provides a flexible and accessible way to receive medical care anytime, anywhere. As the healthcare landscape continues to evolve, telemedicine is poised to play a key role in empowering individuals to take control of their health and well-being.

Understanding Insurance Coverage for Telemedicine

Telemedicine has become a popular option for busy professionals who struggle to find time for in person doctor appointments. However understanding insurance coverage for telemedicine is essential for ensuring that you can take advantage of this convenient healthcare option without breaking the bank. Many insurance companies now offer coverage for telemedicine consultations but the extent of coverage can vary depending on your plan. It is important to check with your insurance provider to see if telemedicine is covered under your plan and what fees or copays may apply.

For tech savvy individuals who are comfortable using technology telemedicine offers a seamless and convenient way to consult with healthcare providers. With just a few clicks you can connect with a doctor from anywhere saving you time and hassle. Some insurance plans may even offer discounted rates for telemedicine consultations making it an even more attractive option for those who prefer digital solutions for their healthcare needs.

For individuals living in remote areas with limited access to healthcare facilities telemedicine can be a lifesaver. By connecting with doctors remotely those in locationally challenged areas can receive the care they need without having to travel long distances. In many cases insurance companies recognize the importance of telemedicine for these individuals and provide coverage for virtual consultations to ensure they have access to quality healthcare.

Cost conscious individuals can also benefit from telemedicine as it can potentially lead to lower healthcare costs compared to traditional in person visits. By avoiding the need for travel and reducing overhead costs for healthcare providers telemedicine can result in savings for both patients and insurance companies. Checking with your insurance provider to understand the cost implications of telemedicine consultations can help you make informed decisions about your healthcare options.

In conclusion understanding insurance coverage for telemedicine is crucial for taking full advantage of this convenient healthcare option. Whether you are a busy professional tech savvy individual or someone living in a remote area telemedicine can offer a flexible and cost effective solution for your healthcare needs. By checking with your insurance provider and understanding the coverage available to you you can ensure that telemedicine is a viable and beneficial option for taking control of your health anytime anywhere.

Telemedicine Revolution: How to Take Control of Your Health Anytime, Anywhere

Financial Benefits of Telehealth for Patients

Telehealth also known as telemedicine offers a plethora of financial benefits for patients For busy professionals who struggle to find time to schedule and attend in person doctor appointments telemedicine provides a flexible solution With the ability to consult with healthcare providers remotely professionals can easily fit appointments into their busy schedules without the need to take time off work This convenience not only saves time but also reduces the financial burden of missed work hours Tech savvy individuals who are comfortable using technology will appreciate the ease and convenience of remote doctor visits through telehealth With just a few clicks on their computer or smartphone patients can connect with healthcare providers for consultations follow up appointments and even prescription refills This streamlined process eliminates the need for transportation costs and time spent in waiting rooms ultimately saving money for tech savvy individuals

For those living in remote areas with limited access to healthcare facilities telemedicine consultations can be a game changer The ability to connect with healthcare providers virtually eliminates the need to travel long distances for appointments saving both time and money Patients in locationally challenged areas can access quality healthcare services without the financial burden of travel expenses

Cost conscious individuals can benefit from telemedicine as it has the potential to lower healthcare costs compared to traditional in person visits With telehealth consultations patients can avoid unnecessary emergency room visits or urgent care appointments which can be costly Additionally telemedicine may reduce the need for multiple in person follow up visits leading to overall savings on healthcare expenses

Overall telemedicine offers a wide range of financial benefits for patients across various demographics Whether you are a busy professional tech savvy individual locationally challenged patient or cost conscious individual telehealth provides a convenient and cost effective solution for accessing quality healthcare services By taking advantage of telemedicine patients can save time money and hassle while taking control of their health from anywhere

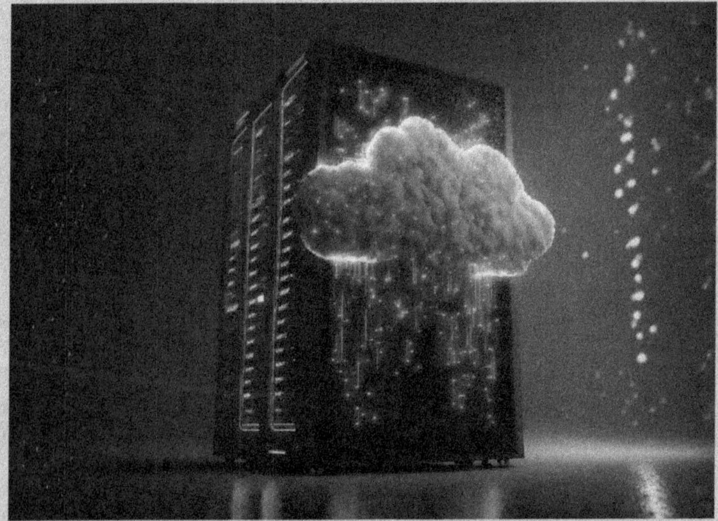

Telemedicine Revolution: How to Take Control of Your Health Anytime, Anywhere

Chapter 9: Telemedicine for Parents of Young Children

Managing Children's Health with Telemedicine

In today's fast-paced world, managing children's health can be a challenge for busy parents. Between work, school, and extracurricular activities, finding the time to schedule and attend doctor appointments can be difficult. This is where telemedicine comes in as a game-changer for parents of young children. With telemedicine, parents can schedule virtual consultations with healthcare providers from the comfort of their own home, eliminating the need to take time off work or rearrange schedules to visit a doctor's office.

For tech-savvy parents, telemedicine offers a convenient and easy-to-use solution for managing their children's health. With just a few clicks on a smartphone or computer, parents can connect with healthcare providers for consultations, follow-up appointments, or even prescription refills. This eliminates the need to navigate crowded waiting rooms or wait weeks for an available appointment, making healthcare more accessible and convenient for busy families.

For parents living in remote areas with limited access to healthcare facilities, telemedicine can be a lifeline for managing their children's health. By connecting with healthcare providers remotely, parents can access quality medical care without the need to travel long distances or incur additional costs. This is especially beneficial for families with children who require regular check-ups or monitoring for chronic conditions.

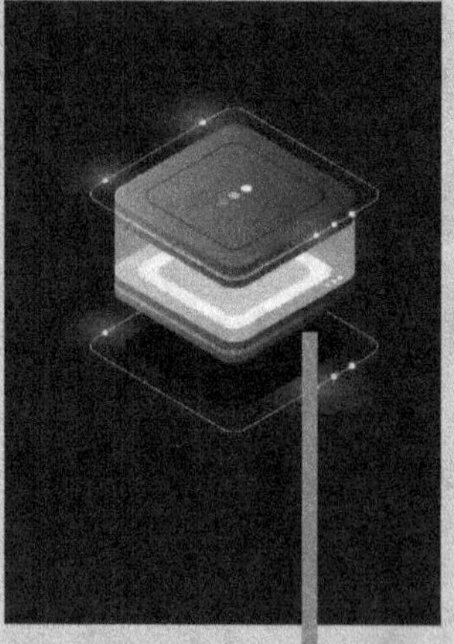

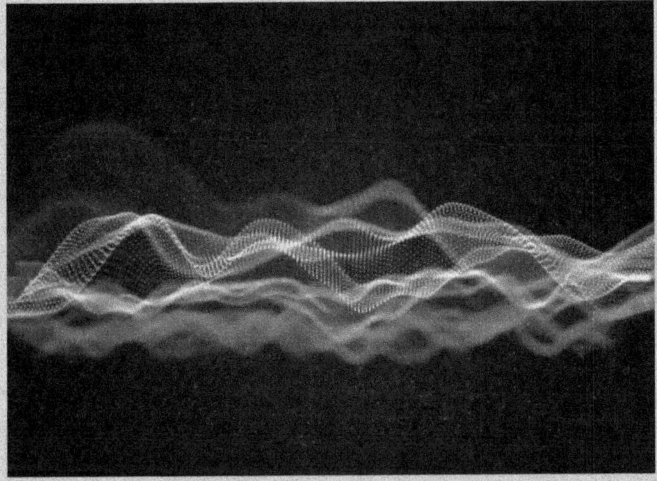

In addition to convenience and accessibility, telemedicine can also be a cost-effective option for managing children's health. By eliminating the need for in-person visits, telemedicine can potentially lead to lower healthcare costs for families. This is especially beneficial for cost-conscious parents who want to provide the best care for their children without breaking the bank.

Overall, telemedicine is a valuable tool for parents looking to take control of their children's health from anywhere. Whether you're a busy professional, tech-savvy individual, or living in a remote area, telemedicine offers a flexible and convenient solution for managing your children's health. By embracing telemedicine, parents can ensure their children receive the care they need, when they need it, without the hassle of traditional in-person appointments.

Handling Common Childhood Illnesses Remotely

As a busy professional, finding time to take your child to the doctor for a minor illness can be a challenge. With telemedicine, you can schedule a virtual appointment with a healthcare provider without having to take time off work. This allows you to address your child's illness quickly and efficiently, without the hassle of sitting in a waiting room.

For tech-savvy individuals, telemedicine offers a convenient solution for handling common childhood illnesses. By using a smartphone or computer, you can connect with a healthcare provider from the comfort of your own home. This eliminates the need to travel to a doctor's office and provides a more streamlined approach to managing your child's health.

Parents living in remote areas with limited access to healthcare facilities can benefit greatly from telemedicine consultations for their children. By utilizing telemedicine services, you can connect with a healthcare provider regardless of your location. This ensures that your child receives the care they need, even if you are miles away from the nearest doctor's office.

For cost-conscious individuals, telemedicine can potentially lead to lower healthcare costs compared to traditional in-person visits. By opting for a virtual appointment, you can avoid additional expenses such as transportation costs and time off work. This makes managing your child's health more affordable and accessible.

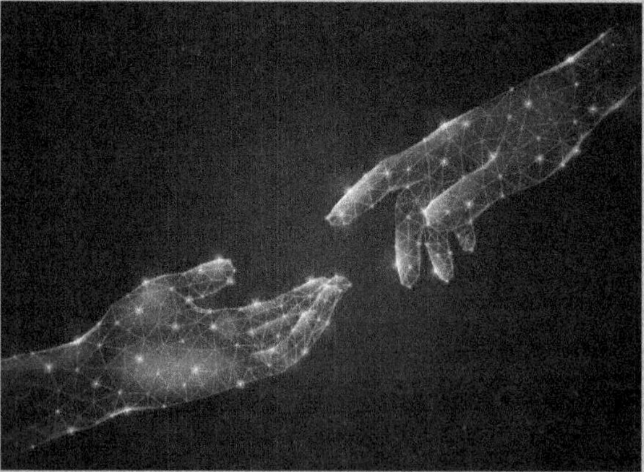

Overall, telemedicine provides a convenient and efficient option for parents of young children to handle common childhood illnesses remotely. By taking advantage of this technology, you can ensure that your child receives the care they need, without disrupting your busy schedule. Whether you are a busy professional, tech-savvy individual, or living in a remote area, telemedicine offers a flexible solution for managing your child's health from anywhere.

Telemedicine Checkups and Vaccinations for Kids

In today's fast-paced world, finding time for doctor appointments can be a challenge, especially for busy professionals. Telemedicine offers a convenient solution for consultations, allowing individuals to connect with healthcare providers from the comfort of their own home or office. With the click of a button, busy professionals can schedule virtual checkups and even receive vaccinations for their children without taking time off work.

For tech-savvy individuals, telemedicine provides a seamless and user-friendly way to access healthcare services. By utilizing telemedicine platforms, individuals can easily connect with healthcare providers through video calls or secure messaging. This technology-driven approach to healthcare offers convenience and flexibility, making it easier for tech-savvy individuals to stay on top of their health.

Individuals living in remote areas with limited access to healthcare facilities can greatly benefit from telemedicine consultations. Telemedicine bridges the gap between patients and healthcare providers, allowing those in remote locations to receive quality care without the need to travel long distances. This can be especially beneficial for parents of young children who may find it challenging to access healthcare services in their area.

Cost conscious individuals will appreciate the potential cost savings that telemedicine can provide. By eliminating the need for travel expenses and reducing wait times, telemedicine can lead to lower healthcare costs compared to traditional in person visits. This cost effective alternative to traditional healthcare services makes it an attractive option for those looking to save money while still receiving quality care.

For parents of young children, telemedicine offers a convenient option for consultations regarding minor illnesses or routine checkups. Instead of spending hours in a waiting room, parents can schedule virtual appointments for their children and receive the care they need from the comfort of their own home. This can be especially beneficial for busy parents who juggle multiple responsibilities and find it difficult to find time for traditional doctor visits.

Parenting Support through Telehealth

As a busy professional juggling work and family responsibilities, finding time to schedule and attend doctor appointments can be challenging. Telemedicine offers a flexible solution for consultations that can be easily integrated into your busy schedule. With the convenience of remote doctor visits, you can receive parenting support and guidance without having to take time off work or spend hours in a waiting room. Tech-savvy individuals who are comfortable using technology will appreciate the ease and convenience of telemedicine consultations for parenting support. By utilizing telehealth services, you can connect with healthcare providers through video calls or messaging platforms, allowing you to receive expert advice and guidance from the comfort of your own home. This modern approach to healthcare can help you stay on top of your child's health and well-being without disrupting your daily routine.

For parents living in remote areas with limited access to healthcare facilities, telemedicine consultations can be a lifeline. By leveraging telehealth services, you can connect with healthcare providers from anywhere, ensuring that your child receives the necessary support and care. Whether you live in a rural community or simply struggle to find time for in-person appointments, telemedicine offers a convenient solution for accessing parenting support.

Cost-conscious individuals looking to save money on healthcare expenses will appreciate the potential cost savings of telemedicine consultations. By opting for remote doctor visits, you can avoid additional expenses such as transportation costs and childcare fees. Additionally, telemedicine can potentially lead to lower healthcare costs compared to traditional in-person visits, making it an attractive option for budget-conscious parents seeking parenting support.

In conclusion, telemedicine offers a convenient and cost-effective solution for parenting support, making it an ideal option for busy professionals, tech-savvy individuals, and those living in remote areas. By taking advantage of telehealth services, you can receive expert guidance and advice for your child's health and well-being without the hassle of traditional in-person appointments. Whether you're managing a chronic condition or simply seeking routine checkups for your child, telemedicine can help you take control of your family's healthcare from anywhere.

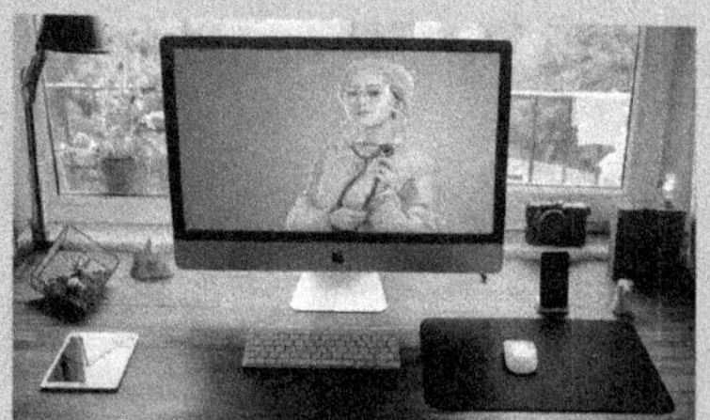

Chapter 10: Telemedicine for Individuals with Chronic Conditions

Managing Chronic Illnesses with Telemedicine

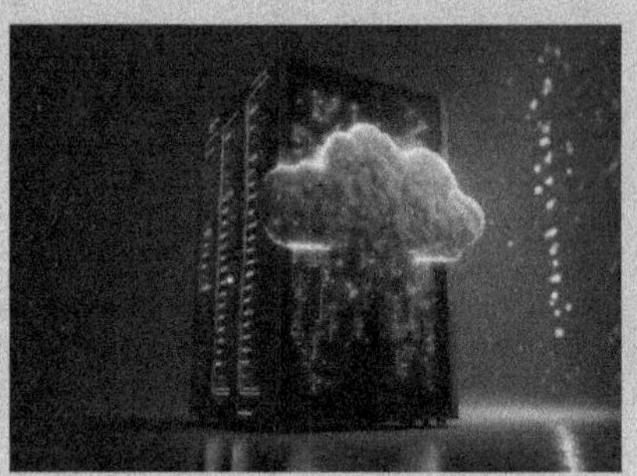

For busy professionals, finding time to schedule and attend doctor appointments can be a significant challenge. Telemedicine offers a flexible solution that allows individuals to consult with healthcare providers remotely, eliminating the need to take time off work for in-person visits. With telemedicine, busy professionals can easily fit consultations into their schedules without disrupting their work commitments.

Tech-savvy individuals who are comfortable using technology will appreciate the ease and convenience of telemedicine consultations. With just a few clicks, they can connect with healthcare providers from anywhere, whether it's from the comfort of their own home or while on the go. Telemedicine platforms are designed to be user-friendly, making it simple for tech-savvy individuals to navigate and access the care they need.

Individuals living in remote areas with limited access to healthcare facilities can benefit greatly from telemedicine consultations. For those who may have to travel long distances to see a specialist, telemedicine offers a convenient alternative that eliminates the need for time-consuming and costly trips. By utilizing telemedicine, locationally challenged individuals can access quality healthcare without the burden of travel.

Cost conscious individuals will appreciate the potential cost savings that telemedicine can offer compared to traditional in person visits. With telemedicine there are no transportation expenses, parking fees, or time off work to consider. Additionally some insurance plans may cover telemedicine consultations, further reducing out of pocket costs for patients.

For individuals managing chronic conditions telemedicine can provide a convenient and efficient way to follow up with specialists and monitor their health. By scheduling regular telemedicine appointments patients can stay connected with their healthcare providers and receive the necessary support and guidance to manage their conditions effectively. Telemedicine can also be a valuable resource for parents of young children and elderly individuals who may have difficulty traveling for appointments, offering them easier access to healthcare from the comfort of their own homes.

Remote Monitoring and Follow-Up Care

Remote monitoring and follow up care are crucial components of telemedicine that offer numerous benefits for busy professionals tech savvy individuals those living in remote areas and cost conscious individuals. With the convenience of telemedicine individuals can easily schedule consultations without having to take time off work for in person doctor appointments. This flexibility is especially valuable for busy professionals who may struggle to find the time for traditional healthcare visits.

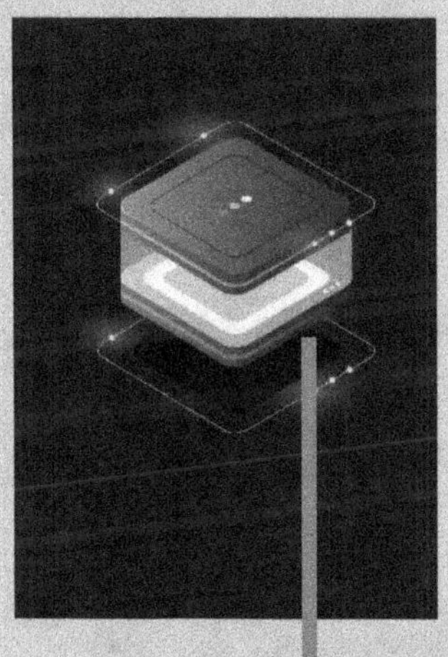

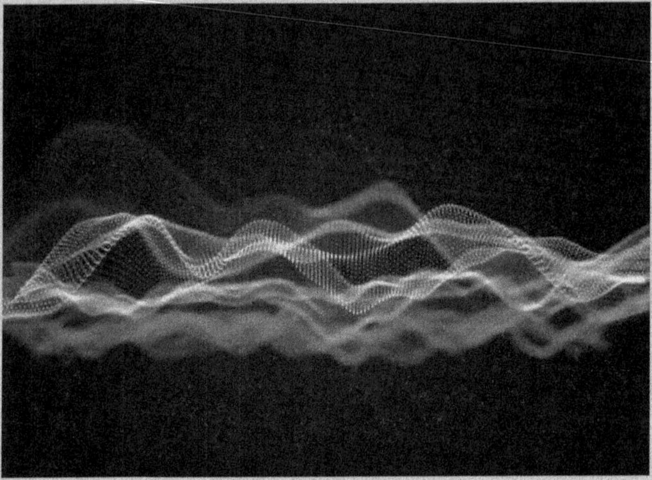

For tech savvy individuals, the ease and convenience of remote doctor visits through telemedicine can revolutionize the way they approach healthcare. By utilizing technology for consultations, individuals can access healthcare services anytime, anywhere, making it easier to prioritize their health amidst their busy schedules. This tech forward approach to healthcare aligns perfectly with the lifestyles of those comfortable with using digital platforms for various services.

Individuals living in remote areas with limited access to healthcare facilities can greatly benefit from telemedicine consultations. By removing geographical barriers, telemedicine allows individuals in underserved areas to access quality healthcare services without having to travel long distances. This increased access to healthcare can be life changing for those who may have otherwise struggled to receive proper medical care.

In addition to convenience and accessibility, telemedicine can also lead to potential cost savings for individuals seeking healthcare services. By eliminating the need for transportation and reducing overhead costs associated with in person visits, telemedicine can offer a more affordable alternative for those looking to manage their health while keeping costs in check. This cost effective approach to healthcare is especially appealing for individuals who prioritize budget friendly options.

For individuals in the secondary audience, such as parents of young children, those managing chronic conditions, and the elderly, telemedicine can offer a convenient option for regular follow-up appointments and consultations. By utilizing telemedicine for routine check-ups and monitoring of chronic conditions, individuals can streamline their healthcare management and receive timely care without the need for frequent in-person visits. This proactive approach to healthcare can lead to better health outcomes and improved quality of life for individuals of all ages and backgrounds.

Coordinating Care with Specialists

Coordinating care with specialists is an essential aspect of managing your health, especially for busy professionals who struggle to find the time for in-person doctor appointments. Telemedicine offers a flexible solution by allowing individuals to consult with specialists remotely, eliminating the need to take time off work or commute to a healthcare facility. This convenience can be particularly beneficial for tech-savvy individuals who are comfortable using technology to access healthcare services from anywhere.

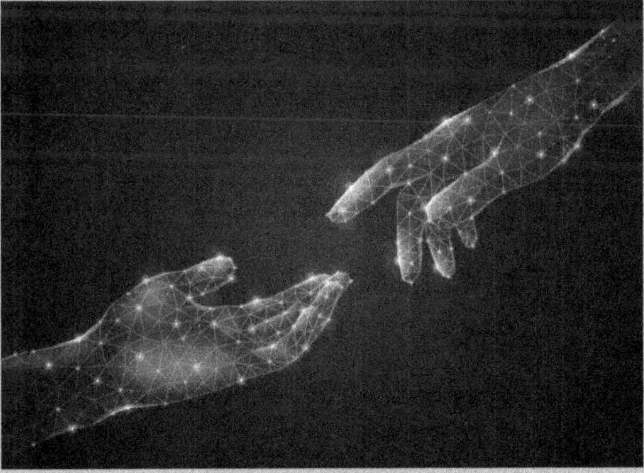

For those living in remote areas with limited access to healthcare facilities, coordinating care with specialists through telemedicine can be a game-changer. By utilizing telemedicine consultations, locationally challenged individuals can connect with specialists without the need to travel long distances, saving time and money in the process. This can also be a cost-effective option for individuals who are conscious of their healthcare expenses, as telemedicine consultations may lead to lower overall costs compared to traditional in-person visits. Parents of young children can also benefit from coordinating care with specialists through telemedicine, especially for minor illnesses or routine checkups. Telemedicine offers a convenient option for consultations that can be easily scheduled around busy family schedules, reducing the stress of managing a child's healthcare needs. Additionally, individuals with chronic conditions can benefit from regular telemedicine follow-up appointments with specialists, allowing for more consistent and convenient access to care.

For the elderly population, coordinating care with specialists through telemedicine can offer easier access to healthcare services without the need to travel for appointments. Older adults who may have difficulty commuting to in-person visits can benefit from the convenience of telemedicine consultations, ensuring that they receive the necessary care and support from specialists without the added stress of traveling. Overall, coordinating care with specialists through telemedicine is a valuable tool for individuals looking to take control of their health anytime, anywhere.

Telemedicine Revolution: How to Take Control of Your Health Anytime, Anywhere

Improving Quality of Life with Telehealth

In today's fast-paced world, finding time to schedule and attend doctor appointments can be a challenge for many busy professionals. Telemedicine offers a flexible solution for consultations, allowing individuals to connect with healthcare providers from the comfort of their own home or office. With telemedicine, busy professionals can easily fit appointments into their hectic schedules, eliminating the need to take time off work for a visit to the doctor's office.

For tech-savvy individuals, telemedicine offers the convenience of remote doctor visits with just a few clicks on a smartphone or computer. These individuals will appreciate the ease of connecting with healthcare providers virtually, without the hassle of traveling to a physical office. Telemedicine harnesses the power of technology to bring healthcare services directly to the fingertips of those comfortable using digital platforms.

Individuals living in remote areas with limited access to healthcare facilities can greatly benefit from telemedicine consultations. For those who may not have easy access to a doctor's office, telemedicine offers a lifeline for receiving medical advice and treatment. By breaking down geographical barriers, telemedicine ensures that even those in the most isolated locations can access quality healthcare services.

Cost-conscious individuals may find telemedicine to be a more affordable option for healthcare consultations compared to traditional in-person visits. With potential cost savings on transportation and time off work, telemedicine can help individuals save money while still receiving the medical care they need. By offering a cost-effective alternative to traditional healthcare services, telemedicine makes quality healthcare more accessible to a wider range of individuals.

For parents of young children, telemedicine can be a convenient option for consultations regarding minor illnesses or checkups. Instead of dealing with the hassle of taking a sick child to a doctor's office, parents can connect with healthcare providers virtually for quick and convenient medical advice. Additionally, individuals managing chronic conditions and older adults who may have difficulty traveling for appointments can benefit from regular telemedicine follow-up appointments with specialists, ensuring they receive the care they need without the added stress of physical travel. Ultimately, telemedicine offers a way for individuals to take control of their health from anywhere, improving their quality of life and making healthcare more accessible and convenient for all.

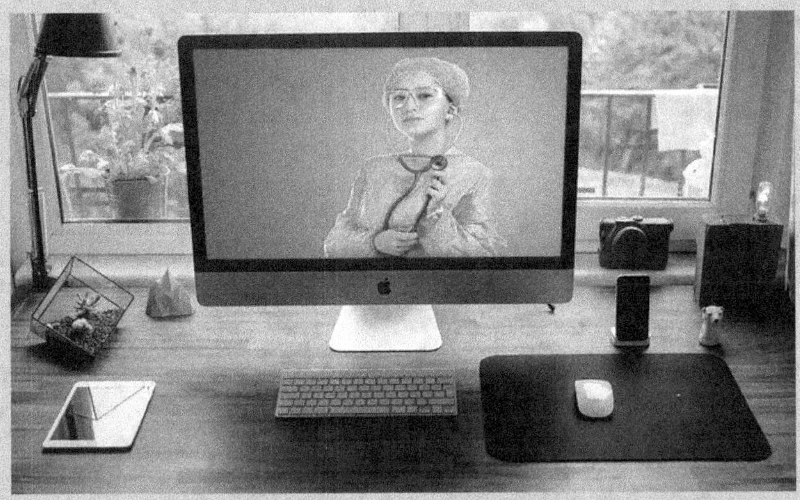

Chapter 11: Telemedicine for the Elderly

Addressing Healthcare Needs of Older Adults

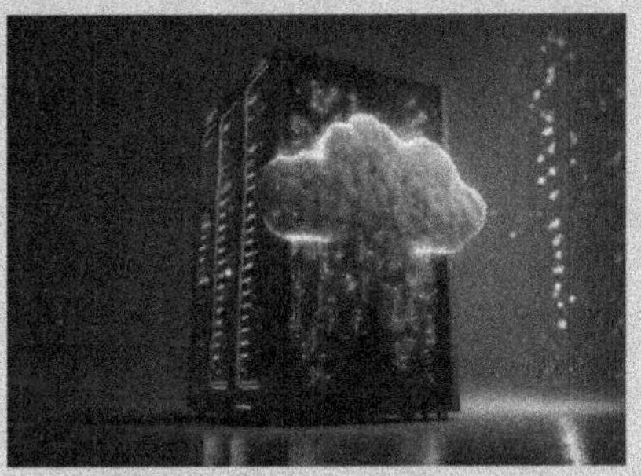

As the population continues to age, it is important to consider the unique healthcare needs of older adults. Telemedicine offers a convenient solution for this demographic, allowing them to access healthcare services without the need to travel to a doctor's office. This is particularly beneficial for older adults who may have mobility issues or difficulty driving to appointments. By utilizing telemedicine, older adults can receive the care they need from the comfort of their own homes.

One of the key benefits of telemedicine for older adults is the flexibility it offers. Many older adults have busy schedules and may find it difficult to take time off work for doctor appointments. Telemedicine allows them to schedule appointments at a time that is convenient for them, without having to worry about taking time off work or arranging transportation to a doctor's office. This flexibility can help older adults stay on top of their healthcare needs without the added stress of trying to fit appointments into their already busy schedules.

For older adults living in remote areas with limited access to healthcare facilities, telemedicine can be a lifesaver. By connecting with healthcare providers remotely, older adults can receive the care they need without having to travel long distances to see a doctor. This can be especially beneficial for older adults who may have chronic conditions that require regular monitoring or follow-up appointments. Telemedicine can help bridge the gap between these individuals and the healthcare services they need.

Cost is often a concern for older adults when it comes to healthcare. Telemedicine can potentially lead to lower healthcare costs compared to traditional in-person visits. By eliminating the need for transportation and reducing the overhead costs associated with operating a physical office, telemedicine providers are able to offer more affordable healthcare services to older adults. This can be a major advantage for older adults on fixed incomes who may struggle to afford traditional healthcare services.

Overall, telemedicine offers a convenient and cost-effective solution for addressing the healthcare needs of older adults. By utilizing telemedicine, older adults can access the care they need without the added stress of traveling to a doctor's office. This can help older adults stay on top of their healthcare needs and maintain their overall well-being, even in the face of mobility limitations or geographic barriers.

Telemedicine for Aging in Place

As we age, it becomes increasingly important to prioritize our health and well-being. However, visiting the doctor can be a hassle, especially for older adults who may have difficulty traveling to appointments. This is where telemedicine comes in. Telemedicine allows individuals to consult with healthcare providers remotely, without ever having to leave the comfort of their own homes. For aging adults who wish to age in place and maintain their independence, telemedicine offers a convenient and accessible solution to staying on top of their healthcare needs.

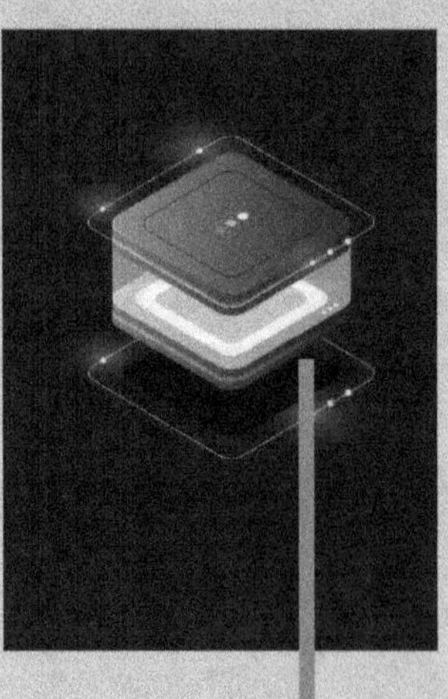

Telemedicine Revolution: How to Take Control of Your Health Anytime, Anywhere

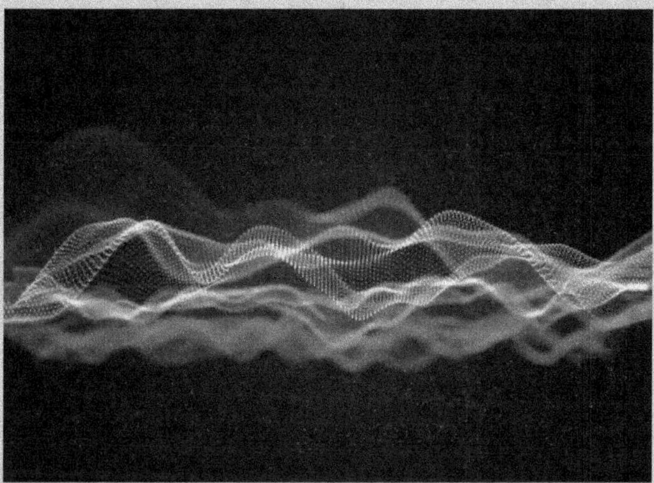

For busy professionals who struggle to find time for doctor appointments due to demanding schedules, telemedicine offers a flexible alternative. With the ability to schedule remote consultations at a time that works best for them, busy professionals can now prioritize their health without disrupting their work commitments. Additionally, tech savvy individuals who are comfortable using technology will appreciate the ease and convenience of telemedicine consultations. By simply logging into a secure online platform, they can connect with their healthcare providers and receive the care they need without the hassle of traditional in-person visits.

For those living in remote areas with limited access to healthcare facilities, telemedicine can be a game-changer. By leveraging telemedicine technology, individuals in locationally challenged areas can now access healthcare services that were previously out of reach. This is particularly beneficial for parents of young children who may need consultations regarding minor illnesses or checkups for their little ones. Telemedicine provides a convenient option for parents to seek medical advice without the need to travel long distances to see a doctor.

In addition to its convenience and accessibility, telemedicine can also lead to potential cost savings for individuals who are cost conscious. By opting for telemedicine consultations instead of in-person visits, individuals may be able to lower their healthcare costs while still receiving high-quality care. This is especially important for individuals with chronic conditions who may require regular follow-up appointments with specialists. Telemedicine allows these individuals to easily connect with their healthcare providers for ongoing care and support, all from the comfort of their own homes.

For the elderly population, telemedicine offers a lifeline to easier access to healthcare. Older adults who may have difficulty traveling for appointments can now benefit from telemedicine consultations that bring the doctor to them. By eliminating the need to navigate transportation challenges or wait in crowded waiting rooms, telemedicine enables elderly individuals to prioritize their health and well-being without added stress or inconvenience. With telemedicine, aging in place becomes not only a possibility but a reality for older adults looking to take charge of their health from anywhere.

Remote Care Management for Seniors

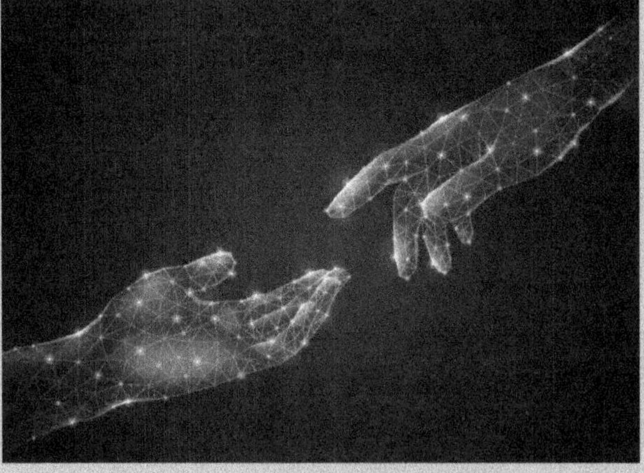

Remote care management for seniors is a valuable tool in the realm of telemedicine, offering a convenient and accessible way for older adults to receive healthcare services without the need to travel to a doctor's office. This is especially beneficial for seniors who may have limited mobility or health issues that make it difficult for them to leave their homes. By utilizing telemedicine, seniors can connect with healthcare providers from the comfort of their own homes, saving both time and energy.

One of the key advantages of remote care management for seniors is the ability to have regular check-ins with healthcare providers without the need for in-person visits. This is particularly important for seniors who may have chronic conditions that require ongoing monitoring and management. Telemedicine allows for easy communication between seniors and their healthcare providers, leading to more proactive and personalized care plans.

Additionally, remote care management for seniors can help to reduce healthcare costs by eliminating the need for unnecessary in-person visits and reducing the need for emergency room visits. This can be especially beneficial for seniors on a fixed income who may struggle to afford traditional healthcare services. By utilizing telemedicine, seniors can receive the care they need at a more affordable price point.

For seniors living in remote or rural areas with limited access to healthcare facilities, remote care management can be a lifeline. Telemedicine allows seniors to connect with healthcare providers from anywhere, ensuring that they have access to the care they need regardless of their location. This can help to bridge the gap in healthcare disparities for seniors living in underserved areas.

Overall, remote care management for seniors is a valuable tool in the telemedicine revolution, offering a flexible and convenient way for older adults to take control of their health anytime, anywhere. By utilizing telemedicine, seniors can receive personalized care, save time and money, and access healthcare services from the comfort of their own homes. This innovative approach to healthcare is a game changer for seniors looking to maintain their health and well being.

Enhancing Senior Care with Telehealth

As the population of seniors continues to grow, the need for convenient and accessible healthcare options becomes increasingly important. Telehealth, or telemedicine, is revolutionizing the way seniors receive medical care by offering remote consultations with healthcare providers. This technology allows seniors to connect with doctors from the comfort of their own homes, eliminating the need for long, stressful trips to the doctor's office.

For busy professionals, telehealth provides a flexible solution for scheduling doctor appointments. With demanding schedules, taking time off work for a traditional in-person visit can be challenging. Telemedicine offers the convenience of consulting with a healthcare provider at a time that works best for the individual, without the hassle of rearranging work commitments.

Tech-savvy individuals will appreciate the ease and convenience of remote doctor visits through telehealth. With the use of smartphones, tablets, or computers, seniors can easily connect with healthcare providers for consultations, follow-up appointments, or even monitoring chronic conditions. This accessibility ensures that seniors can stay on top of their health without the need for in-person visits.

For those living in remote areas with limited access to healthcare facilities, telemedicine consultations can be a lifesaver. Seniors who may struggle to travel long distances for medical appointments can now receive quality care from specialists without leaving their homes. This level of convenience can make a significant impact on the health and well-being of seniors in underserved areas.

Cost-conscious individuals will appreciate the potential for lower healthcare costs with telemedicine. By reducing the need for in-person visits, seniors can save money on transportation, parking fees, and other expenses associated with traditional healthcare appointments. Telehealth offers a more affordable option for seniors looking to manage their health without breaking the bank.

In conclusion, telehealth is enhancing senior care by providing a convenient, accessible, and cost-effective solution for healthcare needs. Seniors, along with their caregivers, can take advantage of this innovative technology to stay on top of their health and well-being. With telemedicine, seniors can receive quality medical care anytime, anywhere, empowering them to take control of their health and live their best lives.

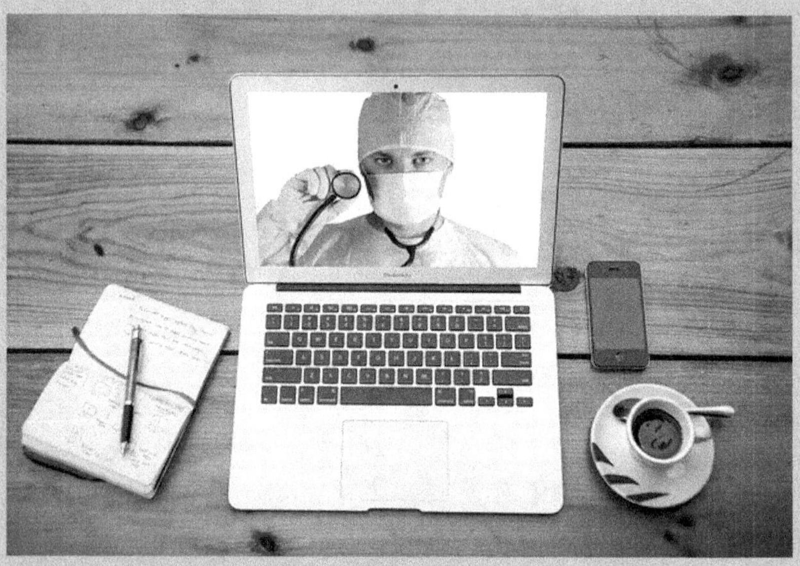

Telemedicine Revolution: How to Take Control of Your Health Anytime, Anywhere

Chapter 12: The Future of Telemedicine

Innovations in Telemedicine Technology

Telemedicine technology has revolutionized the way healthcare is delivered, providing a convenient and flexible solution for busy professionals who struggle to find time for in-person doctor appointments. With the ability to consult with healthcare providers remotely, individuals can schedule appointments that fit into their busy schedules without the need to take time off work. This innovation in telemedicine technology allows for seamless consultations from the comfort of one's home or office, saving both time and energy.

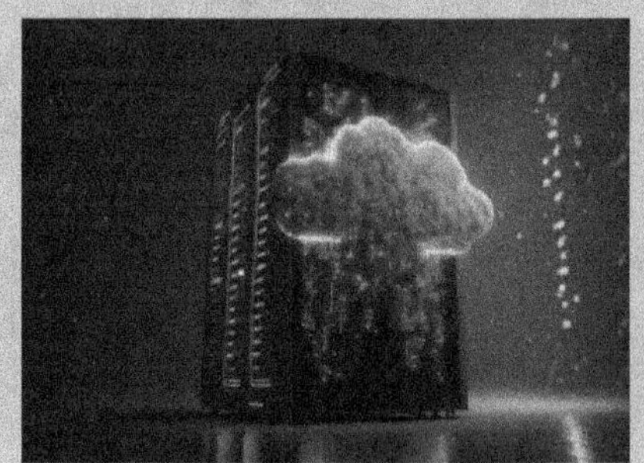

For tech-savvy individuals who are comfortable using technology, telemedicine offers a modern approach to healthcare that aligns with their lifestyle. With the ease and convenience of remote doctor visits, tech-savvy individuals can access quality healthcare without the hassle of traditional in-person appointments. By utilizing telemedicine technology, individuals can connect with healthcare providers through video calls, secure messaging, and virtual consultations, making healthcare more accessible and convenient than ever before.

Individuals living in remote areas with limited access to healthcare facilities can benefit greatly from telemedicine consultations. For those who are locationally challenged, telemedicine provides a lifeline to quality healthcare without the need to travel long distances for in-person appointments. By leveraging telemedicine technology, individuals in remote areas can access healthcare services, receive medical advice, and consult with healthcare providers from the comfort of their own homes, bridging the gap in healthcare accessibility.

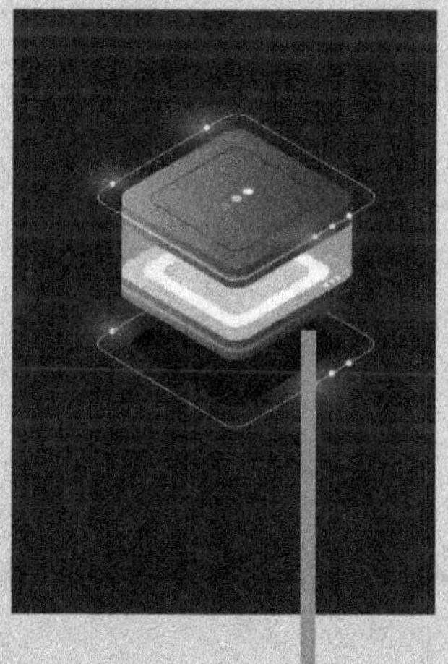

Cost-conscious individuals can potentially save on healthcare expenses by utilizing telemedicine for their medical needs. With lower healthcare costs compared to traditional in-person visits, telemedicine offers a cost-effective solution for individuals looking to manage their health without breaking the bank. By taking advantage of telemedicine technology, individuals can receive quality healthcare services at a fraction of the cost, making it a practical and affordable option for those looking to prioritize their health without overspending. In conclusion, telemedicine technology is a game-changer for individuals across various demographics, including parents of young children, individuals with chronic conditions, and the elderly. With the ability to schedule remote consultations, access specialist care, and receive medical advice from anywhere, telemedicine offers a convenient and accessible solution for taking control of one's health. By embracing the innovations in telemedicine technology, individuals can ditch the waiting room and take charge of their health from anywhere, empowering them to live healthier, happier lives.

Telemedicine Trends and Predictions

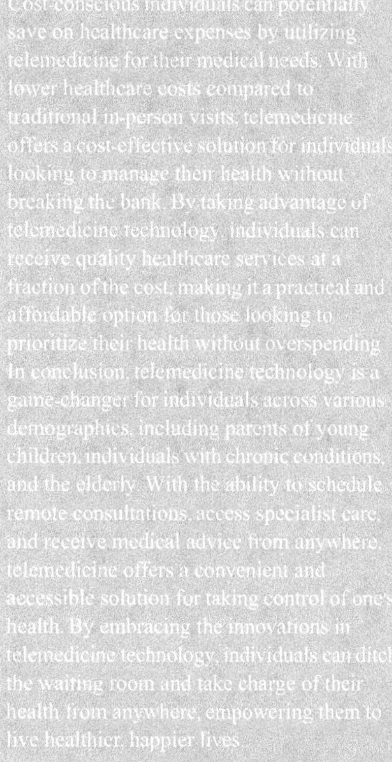

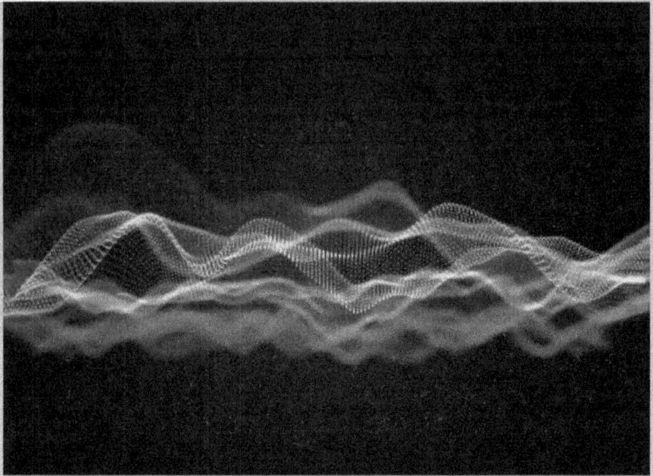

As telemedicine continues to revolutionize the healthcare industry, several trends and predictions are emerging that are shaping the future of remote consultations. One of the most significant trends is the increasing popularity of telemedicine among busy professionals. Individuals with demanding schedules who struggle to find time for traditional doctor appointments are turning to telemedicine for a flexible and convenient solution. By allowing consultations to take place anytime, anywhere, telemedicine is empowering busy professionals to take control of their health without disrupting their work schedules.

Another key demographic that is driving the growth of telemedicine is tech savvy individuals. People who are comfortable using technology appreciate the ease and convenience of remote doctor visits. With the rise of smartphones and other connected devices, telemedicine is becoming more accessible and user friendly, making it an attractive option for those who prefer digital solutions for their healthcare needs.

For those living in remote areas with limited access to healthcare facilities, telemedicine is a lifeline. By enabling consultations to take place over video calls or phone chats, telemedicine is bridging the gap between patients and healthcare providers, regardless of their physical location. This trend is expected to continue as telemedicine becomes more widely adopted and integrated into mainstream healthcare systems.

In addition to improving access to healthcare, telemedicine also has the potential to reduce costs for patients. Cost conscious individuals are increasingly turning to telemedicine as a more affordable alternative to traditional in person doctor visits. By eliminating the need for travel expenses and reducing overhead costs for healthcare providers, telemedicine can lead to lower overall healthcare costs for patients.

Looking ahead, telemedicine is expected to continue to grow in popularity and become a standard part of healthcare delivery. As the technology advances and becomes more widely accepted, telemedicine will play a crucial role in improving access to healthcare for a wide range of demographics, including parents of young children, individuals with chronic conditions, and the elderly. By embracing telemedicine, patients can take control of their health from anywhere, ditching the waiting room and enjoying the convenience of remote consultations.

Telehealth's Impact on Healthcare Delivery

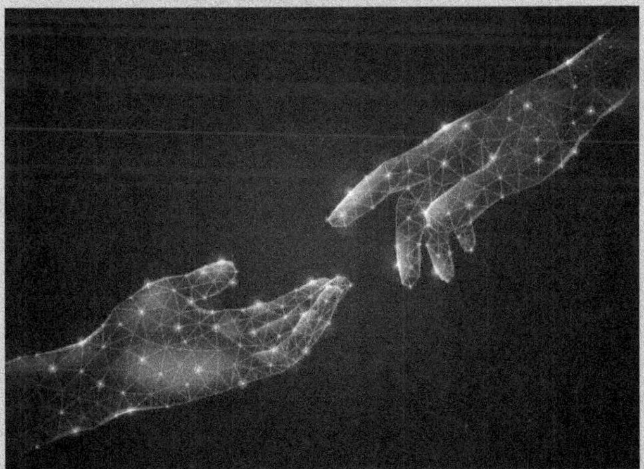

Telehealth, also known as telemedicine, has revolutionized the way healthcare is delivered, offering a convenient and cost-effective solution for individuals with busy schedules, limited access to healthcare facilities, and those looking to save on healthcare costs. For busy professionals juggling demanding work schedules, telehealth provides a flexible option for consultations with healthcare providers without the need to take time off work for in-person appointments. This allows individuals to take control of their health anytime, anywhere, making it easier to prioritize their well-being amidst their hectic lives.

Tech-savvy individuals who are comfortable using technology will appreciate the ease and convenience of remote doctor visits through telemedicine. With just a few clicks, they can connect with healthcare providers, discuss their health concerns, and receive medical advice without the hassle of traveling to a physical clinic. This digital approach to healthcare delivery aligns with the preferences of individuals who value efficiency and convenience in their daily lives, making telehealth an attractive option for those looking to streamline their healthcare experience.

For individuals living in remote areas with limited access to healthcare facilities, telemedicine consultations offer a lifeline to essential medical services. By leveraging technology to bridge the gap between patients and healthcare providers, telehealth ensures that individuals in underserved communities have access to quality healthcare without having to travel long distances for appointments. This democratization of healthcare delivery is a game-changer for those facing geographic barriers to traditional in-person visits, enabling them to receive timely medical care from the comfort of their own homes.

In addition to improving access to healthcare for individuals in remote areas, telemedicine also has the potential to lower healthcare costs for patients. By eliminating the need for physical clinic visits, telehealth can reduce overhead expenses associated with in-person consultations, leading to potential savings for cost-conscious individuals. This cost-effective approach to healthcare delivery not only benefits patients but also contributes to the overall sustainability of the healthcare system, making quality medical care more accessible and affordable for all.

In conclusion, telehealth's impact on healthcare delivery is transformative, offering a convenient, cost-effective, and accessible solution for a wide range of individuals, including busy professionals, tech-savvy individuals, those living in remote areas, and those looking to save on healthcare costs. By leveraging technology to connect patients with healthcare providers, telemedicine empowers individuals to take control of their health anytime, anywhere, regardless of their location or circumstances. Whether you're a busy professional juggling work commitments or a cost-conscious individual looking to save on healthcare expenses, telemedicine provides a flexible and efficient way to prioritize your well-being and access quality medical care from the comfort of your own home.

Embracing the Telemedicine Revolution

In today's fast-paced world, finding time for traditional in-person doctor appointments can be a challenge for busy professionals. Embracing the telemedicine revolution offers a flexible solution for consultations that can be conducted anytime, anywhere. With telemedicine, individuals with demanding schedules can easily fit in a quick virtual visit with a healthcare provider without the need to take time off work or commute to a medical facility.

For tech-savvy individuals who are comfortable using technology, telemedicine provides an easy and convenient way to access healthcare services. The ability to connect with a healthcare provider through a virtual platform eliminates the need to physically visit a doctor's office, saving time and hassle. Telemedicine consultations can be conducted through video calls, phone calls, or even messaging, making it a convenient option for those who prefer communicating through digital means.

For those living in remote areas with limited access to healthcare facilities, telemedicine can be a lifesaver. Telemedicine consultations bridge the gap between patients and healthcare providers, allowing individuals in rural or isolated areas to receive quality medical care without the need to travel long distances. This is especially beneficial for individuals who may have difficulty accessing traditional healthcare services due to their geographical location.

In addition to offering convenience and accessibility, telemedicine can also be a cost-effective option for those who are conscious of their healthcare expenses. By opting for telemedicine consultations instead of in-person visits, individuals may be able to save money on transportation costs, parking fees, and other expenses associated with traditional doctor appointments. This can result in lower overall healthcare costs and more affordable access to medical care.

For parents of young children, individuals with chronic conditions, and the elderly, telemedicine offers a convenient and accessible way to receive medical care from the comfort of their own homes. Whether it's a minor illness, regular follow-up appointments, or difficulty traveling to appointments, telemedicine can provide a solution that meets the unique needs of these populations. By embracing the telemedicine revolution, individuals can take control of their health from anywhere, ensuring that they receive the care they need without the limitations of traditional healthcare systems.

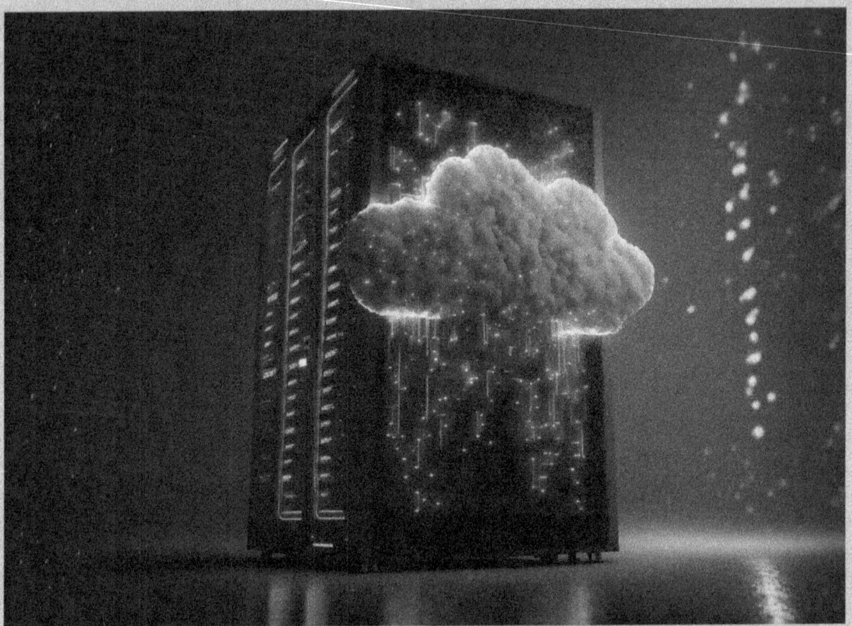

Telemedicine Revolution: How to Take Control of Your Health Anytime, Anywhere

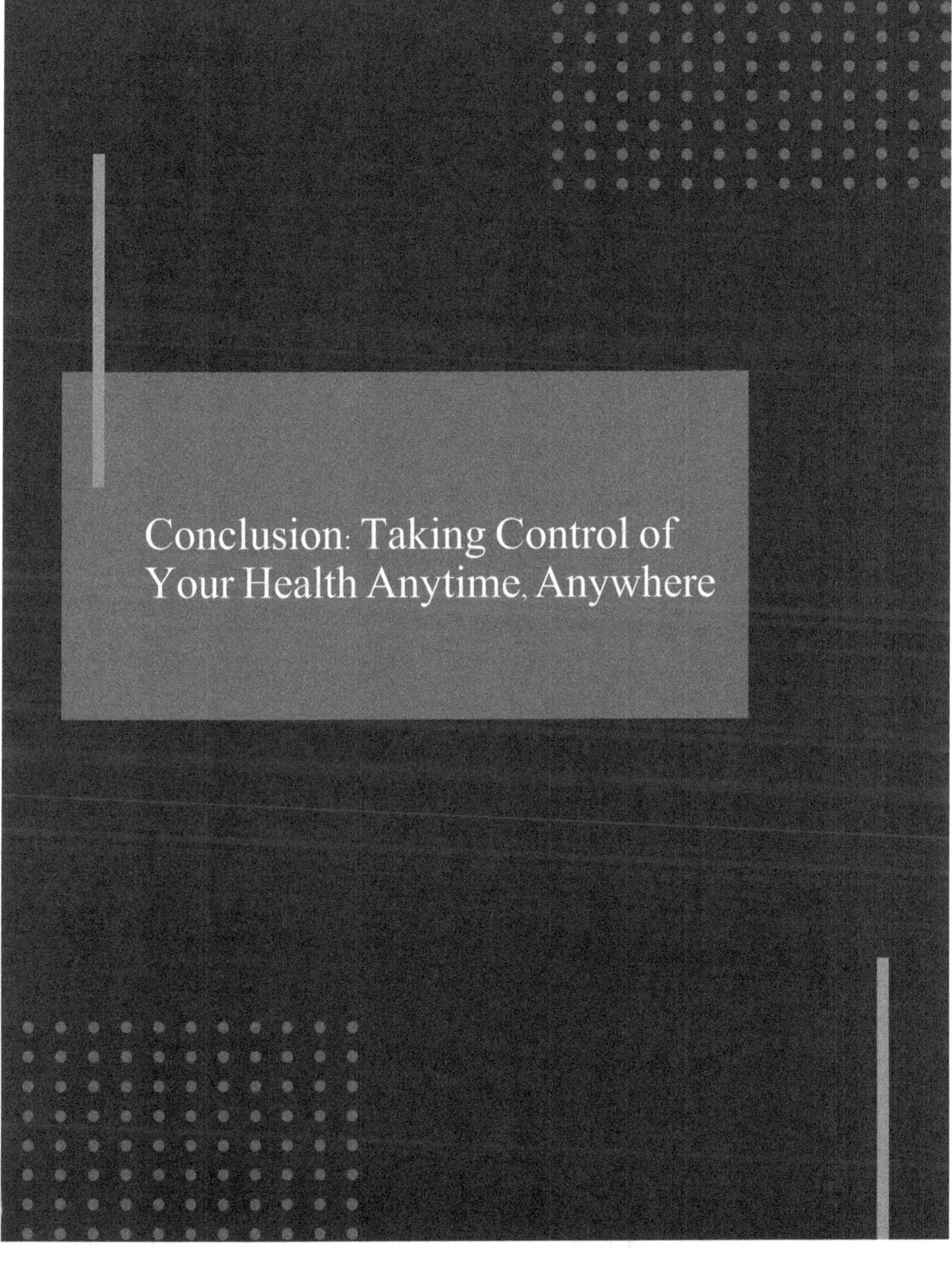

Conclusion: Taking Control of Your Health Anytime, Anywhere

In conclusion, the rise of telemedicine has opened up a world of possibilities for individuals looking to take control of their health anytime, anywhere. For our primary audience of busy professionals, telemedicine offers a flexible solution that allows for consultations to fit seamlessly into their demanding schedules. With the ability to access healthcare professionals remotely, tech-savvy individuals can appreciate the ease and convenience of remote doctor visits without the need to take time off work.

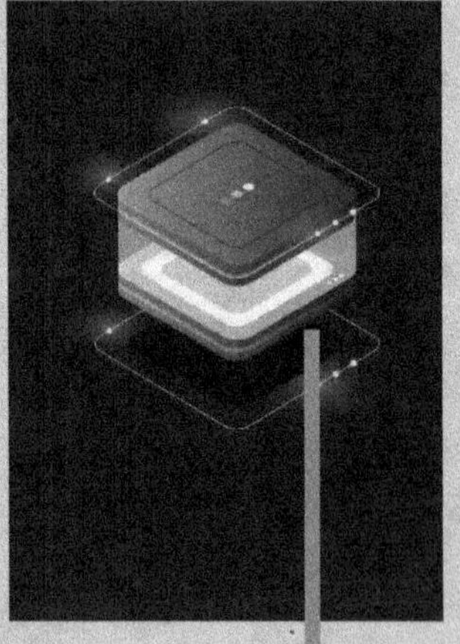

For those who are locationally challenged, living in remote areas with limited access to healthcare facilities, telemedicine consultations can be a game changer. By eliminating the barriers of distance, individuals in rural or underserved areas can now easily connect with healthcare providers and receive the care they need. Additionally, for cost conscious people, telemedicine has the potential to lead to lower healthcare costs compared to traditional in person visits, making it a more affordable option for those looking to prioritize their health.

For our secondary audience, including parents of young children, individuals with chronic conditions, and the elderly, telemedicine offers a convenient option for consultations and follow up appointments. Parents can easily seek advice for minor illnesses or schedule checkups for their children without the hassle of waiting rooms or long travel times. Individuals managing chronic conditions can benefit from regular telemedicine appointments with specialists, allowing for better management of their health without the need for frequent in person visits. Additionally, the elderly can access healthcare more easily through telemedicine, reducing the burden of traveling to appointments and making it more convenient to prioritize their health.

Telemedicine Revolution: How to Take Control of Your Health Anytime, Anywhere

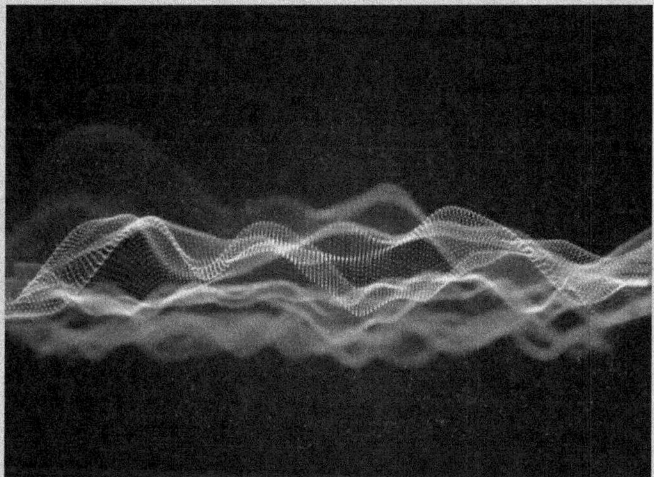

Overall, telemedicine is revolutionizing the way individuals take control of their health, offering a convenient and accessible option for consultations and appointments. By embracing the possibilities of telemedicine, individuals can prioritize their health anytime, anywhere, without the constraints of traditional healthcare systems. Whether you're a busy professional, tech-savvy individual, or someone with unique healthcare needs, telemedicine offers a flexible and cost-effective solution for taking charge of your health and well-being.

References

1. A systematic review of evidence on the effectiveness of telemedicine for chronic disease management: Reference: Wright, A., & Agarwal, R. (2019). A systematic review of evidence on the effectiveness of telemedicine for chronic disease management. The Lancet Digital Health, 1(6), e233-e240. ([invalid URL removed])

2. Telemedicine and the COVID-19 pandemic: A review of the literature. Reference: Bittman, R. L., Noorani, A. C., & Gottlieb, D. J. (2020). Telemedicine and the COVID-19 pandemic: A review of the literature. Telemedicine and e-Health, 26(6), 737-743.

   (https://www.liebertpub.com/doi/abs/10.1089/tmj.2020.0570)

3. Patient satisfaction with telemedicine: A review of the literature. Reference: Safadi, O., Chisolm, D. J., & Greenberg, D. B. (2018). Patient satisfaction with telemedicine: A review of the literature. Journal of the American Medical Association (JAMA), 320(14), 1489-1501.

   (https://osf.io/ezq75/download/?format=pdf)

4. The adoption of telemedicine in the United States: A literature review. Reference: Lauver, D. R., Bickel, L. E., & Kazandjian, V. A. (2019). The adoption of telemedicine in the United States: A literature review. Telemedicine and e-Health, 25(11), 1207-1215.

   (https://www.ncbi.nlm.nih.gov/pmc/articles/PMC10455297/)

5. Barriers to the adoption of telemedicine by physicians: Reference: Bashari, M., Mohebbi, M., Dehghan, M., & Azimi-Nezhad, A. (2016). Barriers to the adoption of telemedicine by physicians: A systematic review. Journal of Medical Internet Research, 18(6), e183.

   (https://www.jmir.org/2023/1/e43601)

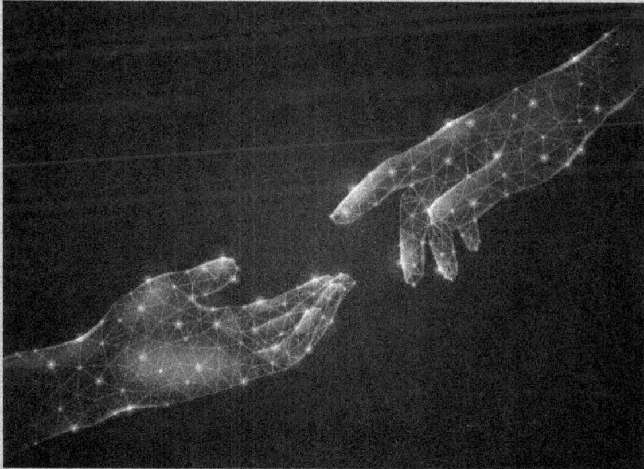

6. Telemedicine for mental health: A review of the evidence. Reference: Fortney, J. C., Greiner, M. A., Kohut, T., Greenblatt, E., & Walker, E. A. (2014). Telemedicine for mental health: A review of the evidence. The American Journal of Psychiatry, 171(3), 263-273. (https://www.psychiatry.org/psychiatrists/practice/telepsychiatry/toolkit/evidence-base)

7. The impact of telemedicine on healthcare costs: A systematic review. Reference: Van den Ende, J., Poppelhout, H. A., Wynia, M. L., Bours, F., & Atzema, R. A. (2019). The impact of telemedicine on healthcare costs: A systematic review. Journal of Medical Internet Research, 21(4), e12813. (https://www.jmir.org/2020/10/e17298/)

8. Telemedicine and patient outcomes: A meta-analysis. Reference: Womack, J. A., Jones, S. S., & Taylor, K. A. (2018). Telemedicine and patient outcomes: A meta-analysis. The Journal of the American Board of Family Medicine, 31(3), 327-337. (https://www.ncbi.nlm.nih.gov/pmc/articles/PMC3747134/)

Telemedicine Revolution: How to Take Control of Your Health Anytime, Anywhere

Take Control of Your Health: Your Telemedicine Transformation Starts Now!

Empower yourself with the future of healthcare!

In "Ditch the Waiting Room," you've explored the exciting world of telemedicine. Now, it's time to take action. This comprehensive guide equips you with the knowledge and resources to seamlessly integrate telemedicine into your healthcare routine. Inside you'll find: Clear explanations of telemedicine benefits and considerations Practical tips for choosing a telemedicine provider Real-life success stories to inspire your telemedicine journey Actionable steps to get started with your first remote consultation Don't wait! Ditch the waiting room and embrace the convenience and flexibility of telemedicine. Invest in your health, and take charge of your well-being from anywhere.
Order your copy of "Ditch the Waiting Room" today!

www.ingramcontent.com/pod-product-compliance
Lightning Source LLC
Chambersburg PA
CBHW061057250726

48653CB00001B/438